T'AI CHI
ACCORDING
TO THE
I CHING

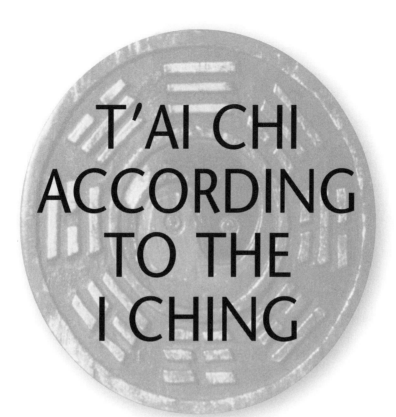

T'AI CHI ACCORDING TO THE I CHING

Embodying the Principles of the Book of Changes

STUART ALVE OLSON

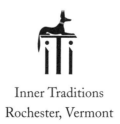

Inner Traditions
Rochester, Vermont

DISCLAIMER

Please note that the author and publisher of this book are NOT RESPON-SIBLE in any manner whatsoever for any injury that may result from practicing the techniques and/or following the instructions given within. Since the physical activities described herein may be too strenuous in nature for some readers to engage in safely, it is essential that a physician be consulted prior to training.

Inner Traditions International
One Park Street
Rochester, Vermont 05767
www.InnerTraditions.com

LIBRARY OF CONGRESS CATALOGING-IN-PUBLICATION DATA

Olson, Stuart Alve.
Tai chi according to the I ching : embodying the principles of
the Book of changes / Stuart Alve Olson.
p. cm.
ISBN 0-89281-944-8 (pbk.)
1. Tai chi. 2. Yi jing. I. Title.
GV504.O48 2001
613.7'148—dc21
2001002883

Printed and bound in the United States

10 9 8 7 6 5 4 3 2 1

Text design and layout by Virginia Scott Bowman
This book was typeset in Caslon with Stone Sans and Kudasai as the display typefaces

There is nothing greater in life than having someone who loves both you and your work.
Thank you, Karen.

Practice without theory is blind,
theory without practice is sterile.

ALBERT EINSTEIN

Contents

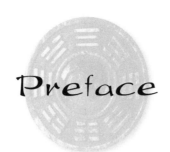

Preface

This book is the culmination of years of study and practice of and interest in T'ai Chi Ch'uan and the I Ching (Book of Changes) and is the last of six drafts produced over the past five years. My focus in this work is on the correlative relationship between the philosophies of T'ai Chi and the I Ching. It is probably the closest to a definitive work on this subject matter in either English or Chinese, yet I do not believe any single book could completely explain the theories and histories of either T'ai Chi or the I Ching. Chinese history is long—very long—with the added problem of historical documents compromised with missing information and many inaccuracies. The philosophical roots of T'ai Chi and the I Ching date back nearly five thousand years to the mythical emperor Fu Hsi, and since that time countless hands have influenced these roots. Considering such historical complications, I made the decision to focus more on the theory and philosophy than on the history of these two subjects, but do provide a general overview of their histories and influences; the correlative material otherwise lacks cohesiveness and clarity.

The "Lotus Stream of Chou" is a Chinese expression referring to the enormous body of philosophical and physiological works created during the ancient Chou period in China and all the materials that either built on those works or were inspired by them. Since the time of Lao Tzu (founder of Taoism) and Confucius, the body of written work produced by the Chinese is staggering and without equal in any other culture. So I hope the reader will appreciate the difficulty in my having to consider and condense the five periods of Chinese history crucial to understanding the influences that now comprise the exercise, a cultural philosophy in motion, called T'ai Chi.

Prior to the Chou dynasty (which began in 1122 B.C.E.), the first period, which is very obscure, dates back to 2852, the time of Fu Hsi, the first emperor of China. In this period of China's history, we also find Huang Ti (2697), the third emperor of China, and a host of early shamans, divinators, and naturalists (Taoists).

The second period comprises the Chou dynasty, in which King Wen, the

Duke of Chou, Lao Tzu, Confucius, and Chuang Tzu provided the works that have influenced all Chinese thinking up to the present times.

In the third period, the era of the pre- and later T'ang dynasties, Chou Tun-i, Chu Hsi, Chung Tung-shu, Chen Tuan, Ko Hung, Lu Tung-pin, practitioners of the Shaolin Kung Fu traditions, and many others helped in clarifying and adding to many of the earlier theories and works of Chinese philosophy.

The Ming dynasty (1368 C.E.), the fourth period, is where we start seeing T'ai Chi take form. In this period, persons critical to T'ai Chi appear, such as Chang San-feng, Wang Tsung, Chang Sung-chi, Wang Chung-yueh, and Chen Wang-ting.

Finally, the Ching dynasty (which began in 1644 C.E.), the fifth period, is when Chen Chang-hsing, Yang Lu-chan, Wu Yu-hsiang, and a multitiered list of masters, lineages, and styles of T'ai Chi appear and when documents pertaining to T'ai Chi became public.

This book tries to keep all these historical eras, personalities, and related works in mind, while trying to be as general and brief as possible.

In the end, this work is probably 90 percent the ideas and works of others and 10 percent mine. No one has ever correlated T'ai Chi to the I Ching satisfactorily, and because of this a great deal of calculating had to be done without a guide. Fortunately, the pieces of the puzzle fit together surprisingly well, and so I can now present what I call *T'ai Chi According to the I Ching*.

The actual process of correlating the I Ching images to T'ai Chi was, in retrospect, far easier than compiling this explanation as to how that was accomplished and how the reader can follow the process. To this end I have provided as much pertinent background material as I thought necessary and have tried my best to match T'ai Chi theoretical aspects with earlier Chinese philosophical treatises and documents. In addition, the work is chronological as best it can be, attempting to take the reader through the developments and influences of both subjects.

I am aware that I touch upon and mention many aspects of T'ai Chi and the I Ching and offer only brief, cursory explanations of them. For this I apologize, but providing extensive explanations to certain ideas and theories would warrant whole books of themselves. Hopefully, this deficiency will cause people to seek further knowledge elsewhere and read the works of other authors.

For those readers who have extensive knowledge of the I Ching, I have purposely excluded such discussions on the theories associated with the ancient

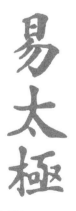

I Ching T'ai Chi

concepts of the Ho and Lo Maps (which are the earlier designs of the Eight Diagrams). I mention this as an example of what was excluded in trying to keep this book focused only on those ideas and concepts relevant to the purpose of this book.

The style of T'ai Chi presented in this book is based on the Yang Style, the most popular system of T'ai Chi practiced in the world today. Although the Yang Style may be the most popular, there really is no standard sequence of movements associated with it. Over the years, many of its greatest teachers have chosen to arrange the postures in various formats. This is why Yang Style forms are sometimes practiced in 24-, 37-, 105-, or 150-posture arrangements. What sets the T'ai Chi form in this book apart from all other T'ai Chi forms is that the 16-Posture I Ching T'ai Chi Form is arranged solely according to the I Ching.

Throughout the book I have most often used the Wade-Giles spelling of Chinese words instead of the modern pinyin system. The title T'ai Chi Ch'uan will often be referred to as T'ai Chi, except in quoting translated texts. All translations are mine.

Acknowledgments

First and foremost, I must thank the late Master Chen Hsin. Without his early work on the I Ching and T'ai Chi contained in his Chinese publication *Chen Style T'ai Chi Ch'uan Illustrated and Explained,* I could never have waded safely through all the theory and conjecture of my own accord.

My heartfelt thanks also go to Master Da Liu, whom I never met, but was a good friend to my teacher, Master T. T. Liang. Liu's book *T'ai Chi and the I-Ching* first sparked my interest in the I Ching and T'ai Chi Ch'uan.

My thanks also to:

Dr. Poon Koon Yui for his many years of distilling Chinese ideas and philosophy and for his unending support and encouragement.

T. T. Liang for his years of instruction and valuable insights to the T'ai Chi classics.

The late Master Jou Tsung-Hwa, whose kind consideration and encouragement led me to begin this work.

Master Soong Jyh-jian, who opened the door into T'ai Chi and the I Ching. His Chinese book, *I Chien Tai Chi Ch'uan,* was very helpful.

My Chinese language and philosophy teacher and good friend, Professor Wu Yi from the Dharma Realm Buddhist University at the City of Ten-Thousand Buddhas. Professor Yi took personal interest in me and taught me I Ching philosophy both in class and in his spare time.

Professor Lin, who many years ago at the City of Ten-Thousand Buddhas gave me the proper tools for approaching and understanding the I Ching beyond divination.

Richard Peterson for his enduring friendship, his exceptional photographic work, and for never letting me think the book was completed just because I wrote it.

Patrick D. Gross for his substantive editing and design work, creating the charts and graphics, and limitless patience while working with me.

The most beautiful of Dragons, Suzanne Lee, for her patience during the T'ai Chi lessons and photography sessions. Her images truly grace the pages of this book.

My student Stan Evers for his interest and persistent encouragement for me to complete this work.

Introduction

The Basis for the Relationship of T'ai Chi and the I Ching

Though it has been established in T'ai Chi classical writings, mentioned in many other works, and hinted at by many teachers, the relationship between T'ai Chi Ch'uan and the I Ching (Book of Changes) has essentially remained a mystery.

T'ai Chi According to the I Ching, however, brings this puzzling relationship into a much clearer light by revealing how the I Ching's Eight Diagram images *(Pa Kua)* relate to the Eight Postures of T'ai Chi, and how in turn they come to form the orderly and proper sequence of the initial sixteen postures of the Before Heaven I Ching T'ai Chi Form. This work also provides corresponding phrases from the *Tao Te Ching (The Classic on the Way and Virtue)* to further establish T'ai Chi's link to the I Ching and classical Taoist philosophy and thought.

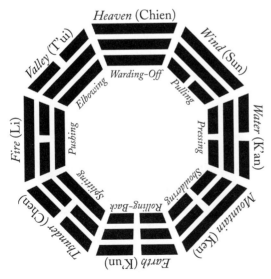

The Eight Diagram images and corresponding Eight Postures

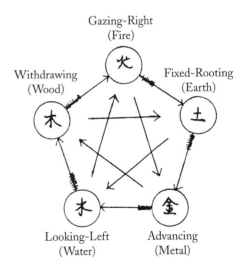

The Five Activities and corresponding elements

1

Since the Eight Diagrams and the corresponding Eight Postures are the very foundation of all T'ai Chi forms, this book provides valuable insights for all T'ai Chi adherents, regardless of the style practiced or the depth of experience. It will also prove invaluable to anyone who has ever studied the I Ching or *Tao Te Ching* and wishes to see how Chinese philosophy can be put into practical use through the art of T'ai Chi Ch'uan.

T'ai Chi draws its I Ching roots mainly from the concluding verses in the *T'ai Chi Ch'uan Treatise*. Considered one of the three major classic and authoritative texts on T'ai Chi theory and practice, the *T'ai Chi Ch'uan Treatise*, presented in its entirety in part 1, clearly establishes the correlations between T'ai Chi and the I Ching in the following excerpt:

> *The Thirteen Postures of Warding-Off, Rolling-Back, Pressing, Pushing, Pulling, Splitting, Elbowing, and Shouldering are known as the Eight Diagrams* (Pa Kua). *Advancing, Withdrawing, Looking-Left, Gazing-Right, and Fixed-Rooting are known as the Five Activities* (Wu Hsing). *Warding-Off, Rolling-Back, Pressing, and Pushing are then* Chien, K'un, K'an, *and* Li—*of the Four Cardinal directions. Pulling, Splitting, Elbowing, and Shouldering are then* Sun, Chen, T'ui, *and* Ken—*of the Four Diagonal directions. Advancing, Withdrawing, Looking-Left, Gazing-Right, and Fixed-Rooting are then Metal, Wood, Water, Fire, and Earth. Joined together they become the Thirteen Postures.*

There has been an ongoing debate as to whether or not these verses were attached to the end of the *T'ai Chi Ch'uan Treatise* and attributed to Chang San-feng simply to lend credence to the idea that a Taoist (San-feng) invented T'ai Chi, thus linking Taoism with T'ai Chi. This theory may hold some weight, but no matter why the verses were included, the facts remain that T'ai Chi and the I Ching do relate and that T'ai Chi's origins and functionings are a development stemming from the I Ching. It *is* curious why the Sung-dynasty Taoist monk, Chang San-feng, is claimed to be the founder of T'ai Chi. His involvement is discussed later, in part 1.

From these concluding verses of the *T'ai Chi Ch'uan Treatise*, the door into the realm and thought of the I Ching as it pertains to T'ai Chi is opened. By knowing that the T'ai Chi posture of Warding-Off is symbolized by Heaven *(Chien)*, Rolling-Back by Earth *(K'un)*, Pressing by Water *(K'an)*, Pushing by Fire *(Li)*, Pulling by Wind *(Sun)*, Splitting by Thunder *(Chen)*, Elbowing by Valley *(T'ui)*, and Shouldering by Mountain *(Ken)*, we can examine T'ai Chi from an entirely new and different perspective.

These verses reveal the building blocks for seeing not only how T'ai Chi correlates to the images of the I Ching, but also how it relates to the ever-present Chinese belief of and adherence to the theory of the Eight Diagrams, which provides a unique key to explaining and understanding T'ai Chi. In fact, even before the Eight Postures of Warding-Off, Rolling-Back, Pressing, Pushing, Pulling, Splitting, Elbowing, and Shouldering were named and specifically linked to the Eight Diagrams, the ideas of the Eight Diagrams were employed and expressed within T'ai Chi—using instead the terms and principles of Adhering, Sticking, Joining, and Following as well as their counterparts of Opposing, Leaning, Discarding, and Resisting. The theories of T'ai Chi are very profound and extensive, created almost entirely from the ancient formulations of the Eight Diagrams, as well as from the incorporated usage of both the T'ai Chi symbol and the attributes of the Five Activities *(Wu Hsing*—Five Elements or Attributes).

The I Ching states that the images must be calculated in the Linear, the Square, and the Circle, which relate not only to the Three Powers' concept of Heaven, Earth, and Man, but uniquely, and most importantly, to the construction, regulation, and expression of T'ai Chi itself. The linear is actually the model whereby the orderly sequence of the T'ai Chi postures are arranged. The square is the model for the regulation of those movements, which in T'ai Chi is called "the square within a circle." The circle is the expression of T'ai Chi. Although all the movements of the postures are constructed and regulated by the linear and the square, they are expressed and performed with circular movements.

For a long time the philosophical correlations between T'ai Chi and the I Ching have been only loosely presented. Within this book the correlations will be made clear by explaining not only why, for example, the image of *Chien* (Heaven) symbolizes the posture of Warding-Off, and so forth, but how positioning the postures in their natural orderly sequence forms the basic movements of the Before Heaven 16-Posture I Ching T'ai Chi Form, and then how stacking these eight, three-lined images upon themselves culminates in the formation of the After Heaven 64-Posture I Ching T'ai Chi Form. I have coined this style of arranging T'ai Chi postures to accord with I Ching images as *I Ching T'ai Chi.*

It is my hope that *T'ai Chi According to the I Ching* will once and for all reveal the concrete underlying relationship between the I Ching, Taoism, and T'ai Chi. For when there is a clear understanding of how the images relate to postures, it becomes ever more amazing as to what the I Ching reveals about the postures themselves. This relationship of T'ai Chi and the I Ching, more than anything else, should elevate T'ai Chi to a completely new level of investigation and consideration, both physiologically and philosophically.

The additional inclusion of corresponding passages from the *T'ai Chi Ch'uan Classics, Tao Te Ching,* and the I Ching gives the work a strong philosophical grounding and can further broaden the understanding of how T'ai Chi is, in fact, a physical expression and culmination of Chinese thought—a logical philosophy in motion.

The first popular English presentation of the I Ching was accomplished by the scholar James Legge, who undertook the enormous and pioneering work of translating this remarkable and ancient text. I can imagine how difficult it must have been for him, not having any previous translations to rely on as references. So when I say that I disagree with some of his translation, it is not a rejection of him or his work, but rather a respectful and minor counter opinion. My main point of disagreement is in his translation of the character for *T'ui,* the ideogram of the seventh diagram, which Legge and those to follow translated as "Marsh" or "Lake," the idea being a symbolic expression of bodies of water, such as oceans, seas, lakes, rivers, streams, or ponds. The character for *T'ui* does include the idea of bodies of water, but it does not refer to the actual substance of water itself. Rather, the meaning of *T'ui* confines itself to where those bodies of water come to rest or where they move through, which is best viewed as the Earth's valleys, hollows, and low places. Thus the reader will see that I have chosen to translate *T'ui* as "Valley."

I support this translation with three main points: (1) The character for *T'ui* literally means "to open up." Again, the idea is of openings as in valleys and channels for water. (2) Each of the Eight Diagrams has its complementary image—such as the images for Fire and Water, Heaven and Earth, Thunder

T'ui
(Valley)

and Wind—but "Bodies of Water" (Marsh or Lake) is not the complementary and opposite image of Mountain; Valley, on the other hand, is. The I Ching itself says that the images of *Ken* (Mountain) and *T'ui* (Valley) are to interchange their influences with each other. A Marsh or Lake is difficult to apply in connection with this injunction, whereas a Valley is a much clearer image for this interchange to be interpreted. (3) In the *Tao Te Ching*, valleys are associated with the perfect behavior of the sage, for the sage emulates the activity of water and seeks the low places that are receptive to all that flows into them. Lao Tzu (a founder of Taoism) also equates the sage with the "Valley Spirit." Valley associates well with Lao Tzu's thought that it is empty spaces that are useful, not the objects themselves. The cup is useful because of its empty space for containing liquid, the window is useful because of its ability to let air and sunlight through it, and the valley is useful for its hollowed out and low aspects because everything flows into it.

Considering all the inferences made to T'ai Chi and the I Ching, one would think many books would already have been written showing this relationship—but I have come across only two in Chinese and one in English that actually attempt to structure their T'ai Chi forms on this correlation. The Chinese book *The Ancestor-Master Chang San-feng's True Transmission on Wu Chi Ch'uan, Illustrated and Explained* by Lu I-su of Hopei province and Ko Tsao Shan of Liao Hui (an ancient state), published in 1935, describes a form that claims to be descended from Chang San-feng. Though it isn't traditional, the 128-Posture Form outlined in that book is adapted to the images of the I Ching. In some ways it appears to be a 32-posture *Chang Ch'uan* (Long Boxing) form quadrupled. It is by far the most cohesive and tangible presentation of the I Ching and T'ai Chi of all the Chinese books I examined. Also, there are a few books on 32-posture *Chang Ch'uan*, but I have never seen one that actually correlates with the I Ching, which is surprising because it would make a perfect match.

The other Chinese book is by Master Soong Jyh-Jian from Taipei, Taiwan. His book *I Chien T'ai Chi Ch'uan*, which appeared in the mid-1960s, is a very serious treatment of the I Ching and T'ai Chi. The form presented contains sixty-four postures, but the actual connection between postures and images is confusing due to the extensive mingling and obscure usages of image manipulation. I am not sure that he really accomplished the goal of connecting the two. But beyond these problems, his knowledge of both the I Ching and T'ai Chi is without question very extensive and well researched. Hopefully, his work will someday appear in English, as it deserves a great deal of attention and examination. I met Master Soong in 1988 and was very impressed with his 64-Posture I Chien T'ai Chi Form and his apparent knowledge and skills. For years after meeting him I mulled the idea of forming I Ching T'ai Chi, as I was so impressed that he also saw the value in presenting a T'ai Chi form that corresponded with the I Ching.

In English there is Da Liu's book *T'ai Chi Ch'uan and I Ching,* published in 1972. Some basic correlations are made, but the majority of the posture and image correlations are derived from just the meaning of the names of the images, not by any logically structured image chronology. The book does contain many valuable insights, however, and should be examined by anyone interested in the subject.

Other T'ai Chi books make the correlation to one degree or another but fail to apply it to the form they present, mentioning the relationship of T'ai Chi to the I Ching as an adjunct theory of T'ai Chi.

It has always struck me as curious why one of the many various styles of T'ai Chi has not been constructed or solely based on a sequence of movements according to the natural changing images of the I Ching. This is odd in that the *T'ai Chi Ch'uan Treatise* itself makes this correlation (as shown in the excerpt on page 2). Numerous books in Chinese include the symbols within their pages but offer no explanations as to why specific images relate to certain T'ai Chi postures. Others devote some explanation to the correlation between T'ai Chi and the I Ching but do not extend these ideas to the arrangements of their forms.

Despite the lack of material showing the T'ai Chi/I Ching relationship through the arrangements of T'ai Chi postures, I drew a great deal of information from the following Chinese sources:

T'ai Chi Ch'uan T'u Chiai (Illustrated Explanation of T'ai Chi Ch'uan) by Chen Hsin. This book contains nearly one hundred pages of I Ching information in connection with T'ai Chi, and is one of the most authoritative books on Chen Style T'ai Chi.

T'ai Chi Ch'uan Chiai I (Explanation of the Meaning of T'ai Chi Ch'uan) by Tung Ying-chieh. His book contains some of the best graphical depictions correlating T'ai Chi with the I Ching.

I realize that T'ai Chi functions perfectly well without the specific construction of arranging T'ai Chi postures according to I Ching philosophy, but I can't help feeling that it is a disservice to not arrange a form to correlate with the I Ching. Why else would the old masters of T'ai Chi have bothered with all the references to the I Ching if they were not going to actually apply it to the sequence of movements?

Why past teachers haven't done this correlating can be explained in a number of ways, ranging from lack of knowledge of the I Ching, to primarily focusing on the self-defense aspects of T'ai Chi, to simply abiding by a form arrangement out of respect to the teacher who taught it. Whatever the reasons, I hope this work will inspire many others to begin practicing T'ai Chi according to the I Ching.

More than anything else, the curious absence of forms showing the relationship of T'ai Chi to the I Ching is what sparked my initial interest. Now that I see the relationship, I have grown ever more curious and amazed at how profound and illuminating this relationship actually is.

T'ai Chi According to the I Ching is as valuable to the I Ching and Taoist reader as it is to the T'ai Chi adherent. Much of the information, especially on the After Heaven and Eight Gates arrangements, is not found in other writings. These arrangements have been misinterpreted and ignored for too long. Herein, however, the I Ching reader will find a great deal of new food for thought. The I Ching, as it is used here, has nothing to do with divination, on which the majority of all I Ching writings base themselves. To that end, this work is a refreshing and new perspective on usage and application. Within the *Ten Wings of the I Ching* it states that there are two purposes or uses of the I Ching—one is for its natural logic, explaining things of the past, and the other is for forecasting, using the I Ching to acquire knowledge of the future. This work follows the first use, natural logic, and shows the calculations of images and correlations of systems already in place.

My presentations on both the history of philosophical influences and related historical figures are far from academic. The purpose of this work has little to do with formal historical presentation and more with the examination of theory—so I hope the reader will forgive the lack of in-depth history. Besides, modern researchers have so many varying views on whether or not the historical figures referred to, such as Fu Hsi, Huang Ti, Lao Tzu, or Chang

San-feng, ever even existed, much less whether they actually wrote anything, that to discuss all their theories would be too painstaking and irrelevant to the purpose at hand.

Whether these persons existed or not, or whether they actually wrote anything or not, is really unimportant. What is important is that certain works and philosophies do exist and have provided great value to the development of Chinese culture. The Chinese, in fact, have no conscious problem or guilt in creating mythical founders for teachings they have embraced as truth. Whether that founder really existed or not makes little difference to them. The inspiration and symbolism derived from such creations do, however, mean a great deal. The creation of "Wild History," as the Chinese call it, can sometimes be more valid and useful than vague and undetermined history.

I sincerely hope that this presentation will not only provide a clear description of the relationship between T'ai Chi and the I Ching, but will also prove philosophically intriguing as well. For as much influence as the I Ching has had on T'ai Chi, Taoism and Taoist philosophy have had an equal role. So by the inclusion of comparative Taoist verses from the *Tao Te Ching* with those from T'ai Chi and I Ching texts, I hope that the reader will be even further enriched by this material.

PART I

The Undercurrents of I Ching T'ai Chi

1 T'ai Chi

A system of exercise based on adapting to change yet embracing the fixed, like a willow tree whose branches sway easily in the wind while its trunk and roots remain unmoved, T'ai Chi Ch'uan—Supreme Ultimate Boxing (simply referred to as T'ai Chi)—is without question a national treasure to the Chinese. The philosophies inherent and adapted to T'ai Chi have undeniably altered many of the behaviors and outlooks on life for the Chinese—for T'ai Chi is the very physical expression and culmination of Chinese philosophy, thought, and practice developed in more than three thousand years of history.

There is no solid evidence of its true origin, nor does it appear to be the invention of a single person or group of persons, nor is there one standard way in which to either describe or practice it. The only certainty about it is that it is very popular within and without China. A testament to its Chinese popularity is what you can witness early mornings at any park or available empty space along China's streets—hundreds of people moving slowly to the rhythms of T'ai Chi movements.

Chinese T'ai Chi adherents have developed a quiet philosophy about these early morning vigils of slowness and quietude. They believe that starting their days with slow, methodic movements, mental tranquillity, and harmonious breathing will influence their daily activities to proceed smoothly and be void of tension. In the West we wake up and begin the stimulation process to jolt our way into the day with coffee, cigarettes, television, radio, a quick breakfast, fighting congested traffic to our workplaces; it is no wonder we suffer so many maladies due to tension and anxiety. Despite our enormous health care, insurance, and research institutions, the West still suffers the highest incidence in the world of illnesses and diseases relating to tension and anxiety. Arthritis, heart disease, high blood pressure, ulcers, blood impurities, and cancer run rampant in our population. We have made a great error in trusting others, namely the medical world, for the maintenance of our health. It is imperative that we take responsibility for our own well-being.

We in the West have long considered the body to be like a car. When it breaks we bring it to the mechanic and hope that it can be repaired. The

Chinese, on the other hand, learned long ago that the body is like a garden that must be weeded, nourished, and well tended. The West has been clouded by the curative approach to health—we wait until we get sick before seeking to care for ourselves. The Chinese take the preventative route, using natural methods in order to avoid illness. T'ai Chi has long been a staple medicine to that end.

The most basic reason for undertaking the practice of T'ai Chi is simply to increase your sense of well-being and health. This comes about from adhering to the proper application of the principles that govern correct movement within T'ai Chi. When practicing T'ai Chi properly, three main benefits are experienced: (1) increased blood circulation, which produces greater body heat and makes you feel more active and alert; (2) the breath sinks low into the abdomen, which stimulates the *ch'i* (the vital energy of the body), bringing about a greater sense of strength and vitality; (3) increased sense of central equilibrium—since the movements depend on rooted movement in conjunction with the breath, the entire sense of balance is greatly heightened. There are many other benefits, but these three are the most apparent to T'ai Chi adherents who practice correctly.

T'ai Chi is considered by the Chinese to be a soft martial art. It has sometimes been referred to as "cotton-fist boxing" or "shadowboxing." The idea that T'ai Chi is a "soft" martial art, however, is inaccurate. Although its movements may appear soft, in expression of its applications the energy derived is quite strong. The T'ai Chi Ch'uan Treatise says, "The arms are like an iron bar wrapped in cotton." The premise of T'ai Chi is that the underlying principle of movement is slow and relaxed, with movements generated from the waist and legs. Movements generated primarily from the arms and shoulders are seen in the harder styles of martial arts such as Japanese Karate, derived from Shaolin Kung Fu Boxing and made famous by Buddhist monks of the Shaolin Kung Fu Temple.

T'ai Chi is a very rich art in that the purposes and benefits of its practice are multifold. In the main, it is a health art, commonly called "nourishing life art" *(yang sheng shu)* by the Chinese. Its ability to stimulate blood flow, relieve the body of stress and tension, and relax the muscles is quite well known among all its practitioners. It is undoubtedly one of the best forms of *ch'i kung* (skillful breathing) practices and developments, as the entire body must move in unison with the breathing and all the attention is placed in the lower abdomen (*tan-t'ien*, "Field of Elixir"). Also, it is an extremely effective means of self-defense, but not in the sense of mainstream martial arts like Karate or Kung Fu. T'ai Chi makes use of many *intrinsic* skills against an opponent, such as Yielding, Following, Adhering, Enticing, Borrowing, and so on. In Chinese thought, T'ai Chi expresses the use of *chin* (intrinsic energy), which is like the energy produced from employing a whip. Shaolin Kung Fu expresses the use of *li* (external muscular force), which is like that of striking with a stick. T'ai Chi also maintains an attitude of playfulness, reaction force, and pliability during an attack, and Shaolin Kung Fu unyieldingness, speed, and strength. The term "self-defense" in regard to T'ai Chi can also be misinterpreted, because it does not apply in its ultimate sense of fighting. Self-defense is meant more to indicate "defense against the self." It is our own selves who make mistakes, our own clumsiness, errors in judgment, lack of awareness and mindfulness that cause us to get hurt, whether that be by a fall from losing our balance or in reacting poorly when being attacked in a fight.

Another aspect of T'ai Chi practice is the development of wisdom, or mental accomplishment. When a person focuses his or her mind on the principles of Yielding, Relaxing, Adhering, and so on, these aspects then, over time, also become part of the person's temperament, bringing forth a more tranquil and less aggressive response to the obstacles in life. It also implies the attainment of *Shen Ming* (Illumined Spirit), developed from the heightened skills of Interpreting Energy (one of the intrinsic energies that T'ai Chi training develops). *Shen Ming* may also be defined as a very exalted stage of perspective awareness.

T'ai Chi also extends to the goal of longevity and immortality. Briefly stated, T'ai Chi practice enables increased stimulation of blood flow, an increased sense of well-being, and a tranquil body and mind. These are the very catalysts for bringing someone into old age with glowing health, which the Chinese call "youthfulness within old age." In the Chinese view, old age is wonderful providing you have health. Without health even your youth can be pure misery. So the achievement of longevity is sought for the reasons of acquiring a comfortable and healthy old age.

In acquiring longevity, a great deal of attention is likewise paid to achieving immortality *(hsien)*. To the Chinese this term has various meanings. The most accepted view is that immortality allows you to depart from this world fully conscious, with your spirit intact. The process for this begins first with increasing your blood flow, for within the blood is the inherent oxygen, *ch'i* (vital energy and/or breath). *Ch'i* is like the steam coming forth from boiling water. When the blood is stimulated, it becomes warm. This warm blood heats the sinews and tendons, and from there the heat and moisture penetrate and collect in the bones, thus producing marrow. This same process of heating the blood gathers the *ch'i* into the *tan-t'ien* (Field of Elixir), which then spreads throughout the meridians and collaterals of the body, circulating the *ch'i* to and from the *tan-t'ien* so that it can congeal into the Pill of Immortality. Mobilizing the *ch'i* and congealing it in the *tan-t'ien* refines it into an elixir of sorts that then reportedly renders a person immortal.

In essence, the purpose of T'ai Chi, not unlike all Taoist practices, is to restore your bones and muscles to the pliability of those of a child, to restore your breath into your abdomen, and to empty the mind of all anxiety and negative impulses. Positively affecting your body, breath, and mind opens the very gateways to not only acquiring optimum health and longevity, but immortality as well.

A very old and common adage in China is *Chang Sheng Bu Lao,* which literally translates as "long life but not old." More correctly its meaning is

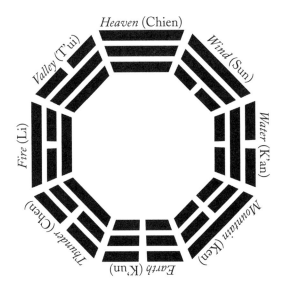

The Eight Diagrams symbolize all the phenomena in our world and are known collectively as the Before Heaven images.

"youthfulness within old age." To have health within one's senior years is of utmost importance to the Chinese, and everything else is secondary. Without health, much less can be accomplished and a person's ability to enjoy old age is greatly reduced. T'ai Chi has long been a primary means for seeking this goal of being youthful in old age.

Generally speaking, nothing in China has much worth unless it is old and has proven itself with the test of time. In the West, it is the new and quick that get our undaunted support, and the old is discarded as outdated. In the T'ai Chi classical writings there is a verse that serves well in changing one's attitude about overvaluing youth and swiftness. The verse states, "If you see an old man withstanding many opponents, what has this to do with swiftness?"

When I was in my thirties and studying T'ai Chi with Master T. T. Liang, who was in his eighties, I was frequently humbled by how easily he would defeat me in any sparring exercise. My culture had taught me that youth, speed, and strength were superior, but I soon learned that these were my catalysts for defeat. Master Liang proved time and time again that internal strength was far greater than external, that yielding overcomes the unyielding, and that calmness and concentration always surpass aggressiveness and anxiousness.

In the ancient book of *Chuang Tzu* is a story about a prince who needed to get to an outpost quickly, as war with a neighboring kingdom was imminent. He boarded his carriage and the driver sped off, whipping the horses to move as quickly as possible. The prince stuck his head out the carriage door and yelled to the driver, "Slow up, slow up! I am in a hurry." This story shows that if we go too fast we run the risk of breaking down and never getting there at all. This idea of taking one's time, more than any other concept, has permeated Chinese thinking and is the attitude that underlies all of T'ai Chi practice in Chinese culture.

2   The Eight Diagrams and the I Ching

The *Pa Kua* (Eight Diagrams) are as old as Chinese culture itself, dating back nearly five thousand years and were supposedly invented by Fu Hsi, the mythical first emperor of China (2852 B.C.E.).

The Eight Diagrams are in essence the first computerlike oracle program for determining the changes occurring in the Heavenly, Earthly, and Humanly realms—acting as a visual imagery indicator of past, present, and future conditions and events. Fu Hsi's invention of the Eight Diagrams was a very enlightened and profound discovery that has been instrumental in the formation of Chinese culture ever since. These eight simple three-lined images symbolize every aspect of the macro and micro orders of the material and immaterial realms of existence. Developed over a long period of time by numerous sages and scholars, the myriad Eight Diagram theories are so broad and extensive that to explain them in detail would mean having to describe Chinese culture itself from the beginning.

The Eight Diagrams existed in their original form, as a distinct system of divination and archetype for divining wisdom, for nearly three thousand years. Emperor Fu Hsi claimed to have seen eight three-lined images on the back of a tortoise shell or on the back of a Dragon-Horse that flew out of the Yellow River—the legends differ throughout different periods of time. Some accounts have Fu Hsi as the visionary of the Ho River Chart and Emperor Shen Nung, the second of the Five Legendary Emperors (2000–1700 B.C.E.), of the Lo River Chart (see pp. 22–23 for an explanation of the Ho and Lo arrangements, which are the earlier designs of the Eight Diagrams). The markings on the shell appeared as a series of dots. From this vision developed the theory of the Eight Diagrams, which later led to the I Ching itself.

The most drastic changes came about when the founder of the Chou dynasty, King Wen (1171–1122 B.C.E.), and his son, the Duke of Chou (died 1094 B.C.E.), formed what we now know as the I Ching. Taking the Eight Diagrams, King Wen stacked each image upon itself and upon each other, making sixty-four images, which have been commonly and erroneously called hexagrams (a hexagram is a six-sided image, not six stacked lines). King Wen also wrote a *tuan ch'uan* (textual explanation) on each of the sixty-four images. It is also supposed that the creation of the sixty-four images dates farther back into the Shang dynasty, or that Fu Hsi had created them himself. King Wen's other great contribution to the formation of the I Ching was his creation of the After Heaven arrangement of the Eight Diagrams, which he redesigned from an earlier chart of the Ho and Lo River Charts. This arrangement, in part, serves as an inner reflective view of the Before Heaven arrangement (which symbolizes all the phenomena in our world). The Duke of Chou, while imprisoned (his father lost the empire but later regained it), compiled the *Yao Tz'u*, the textual interpretations of the individual six lines for each of the sixty-four images. Through them the I Ching had found its lasting form.

About five hundred years later Confucius (Kung Fu Tzu, born 551 B.C.E.) and some of his various disciples added commentaries to the I Ching, calling them the Ten Wings, which are the ten textual divisions or commentaries on the three primary sections of the I Ching—the sixty-four images *(Kua)*, the text on the images *(Tuan Ch'uan)*, and the text on the lines *(Yao Tz'u)*. All of these works combined are what we presently know as the Book of Changes (I Ching)—sometimes called the Book of Chou.

Since the time of Confucius, various Taoist, neo-Confucian, and Buddhist interpretations of the I Ching started to appear. About fifteen hundred years after Confucius and his disciples wrote their commentaries, the neo-Confucianists Chou Tun-i, Chu Hsi, and Chung Tung-shou all contributed greatly to the ideas of T'ai Chi, *yin* and *yang*, the Five Activities, and the Eight Diagrams. Chou Tun-i and Chu Hsi wrote very important treatises that helped clarify the "Supreme Ultimate," the philosophy of the T'ai Chi symbol.

Chinese philosophy could not have developed in the manner it did without the great academic works of Confucians and neo-Confucians. Taoism itself owes greatly to the works of Confucian scholars, and, in fairness, they owe the Taoists as well. Most neo-Confucians, whether by accident or choice, seemed to write with a bent toward Taoist ideals. We must keep in mind and give credit to the Confucians, for they were the active scholars of Chinese philosophy, while Taoists for the most part were the active non-doers of academic writings.

The I Ching has enthralled readers since its early days up to the present. It is the very basis for understanding *yin-yang* theory—the interaction of opposite forces in nature, both on the level of the microcosmic and macrocosmic.

History records that there were once two other divinational books similar to the I Ching—the *Kwei Tsang* and *Lien Shan*—which reportedly also used eight images as their foundation for divination. These three books were supposedly used for the separate matters of divining human affairs, such as governing, military strategy, divination, medicine, and spiritual matters. The *Kwei Tsang* and *Lien Shan* are lost to us, however, and are only mentioned in a few historical records. Luckily, during the great book burning by the Emperor Huang Ti of the Chin dynasty (died 209 B.C.E.) the I Ching was saved, as he considered it worthwhile for his newly unified China.

It would be virtually impossible to gauge the influences that the I Ching and its basic components of the Eight Diagrams have had on Chinese culture and history. History records that almost every emperor sought the use of the I Ching for both military and governing concerns. In China, religion, philosophy, medical-health practice, fortune-telling, *feng shui*, geomantic divination, astrology, folklore magic beliefs, mystical and alchemical sciences, and more developed from, adopted, or integrated in some manner ideas inherent to the Eight Diagrams and the I Ching. They permeate the entire undercurrent of Chinese civilization, philosophy, and culture.

Presently, the Eight Diagrams are widely used throughout Asia as a means of warding off evil spirits and calamities. Written on ocher paper, the diagrams act as a talisman, or as plaques, hung over doorways and windows to keep evil influences away. There are few homes and businesses in Asia that do not display one or more of these various symbols.

It is believed that these eight symbols are auspicious and bring good fortune to those who bear them. In South Korea, the Four Emblems (derived from the *Pa Kua)* are seen in its flag along with the T'ai Chi double-fish emblem. There are few temples (Buddhist, Taoist, and Confucian alike) that do not have a divinational forecasting shrine to which the populace can come to divine their future—and all the methods used derive in some manner from the Eight Diagrams. Along the streets leading to the temples, fortune-tellers, divinators, and astrologers are also using methods that incorporate principles inherent to the Eight Diagrams.

When a male child is born, for example, his destiny *(ming)* is determined by calculating the year, the month (or moon), the day, and the hour in which he was born. These four calculations are each represented by a diagram, and from these four diagrams, two six-line images are constructed that determine his I

Ching Life Symbols for both his Before and After Heaven destinies.

According to the *Nei Ching*, a work attributed to the Yellow Emperor, Huang Ti, a male child is ruled numerologically by the number eight. He is said to develop his milk teeth at eight months, losing them during his eighth year. When he turns sixteen (2 x 8) he has become a man because he is capable then of reproducing himself. At thirty-two (4 x 8) he will have set his destiny and ends his Before Heaven years of life. At sixty-four (8 x 8) he either benefits or suffers from how he managed his After Heaven years, and at this stage of his life is no longer interested in reproduction.

These four stages coincide with his four birth images as well. For example, a male child could be born in the year of the Dragon, in the moon of a Tiger, the day of a Rooster, and the hour of a Dog. These four animal signs can each then be interpreted as to the destiny of the person, and further be associated to specific diagrams and images of the I Ching, for both his Before and After Heaven years of life.

A female child, however, is ruled by the number seven, but the relation to the Eight Diagrams remains the same. At seven months she acquires milk teeth, and at seven years she loses them. At fourteen she is a woman, at twenty-eight her Before Heaven years are being completed, and at forty-nine she benefits or suffers according to her After Heaven destiny. The only difference in the male/female descriptions is that a male is considered sexually potent at sixteen and the female at age twenty-eight. That is a twelve-year difference, one complete astrological cycle apart. This is one reason that in early China, especially in families of wealth or position, marriages were considered best arranged when the male was one astrological cycle ahead of the female in age. However, there could be good same-cycle marriages arranged as long as the couple's ages did not fall below an eight-year difference.

Another important reason marriages were considered better between older men and younger women was that the older man had time to finish his studies and become financially secure before taking a wife. For the female, it meant entering into a new family in which the husband was mature and could care for her and their children's needs, without all the beginning struggles of same-age marriages. All of these ideas on marriage were originally calculated and viewed from the theories contained within the Eight Diagrams and the I Ching. Ever since the takeover by Mao Tse-tung, however, the practice of arranged marriages has been almost entirely eradicated from Chinese life.

Since the I Ching and its Eight Diagram images are seen as representing all phenomena, a link can be established between the I Ching and modern scientific theory. Scientists have reported that DNA has thirty-two basic building blocks and that these likewise contain (+) male and female (-) components (two amino acids), another way of equating *yin* and *yang*. Also, in attempting to annihilate certain subatomic particles, scientists discovered that the particles would simply re-create an opposite likeness of themselves, what quantum physicists call "daughter cells." This discovery of daughter cells relates to the ideas on *yin-yang* theory developed from the Eight Diagrams. When *yin* or *yang* reaches its extreme it will become its opposite, and the process of change continues.

Despite the fact that my comparison here isn't scientifically adequate, the notion that the numerological building blocks of the human race relate exactly to the numerological building blocks of the I Ching is at once staggering and exciting. The I Ching has sixty-four primary images, of which thirty-two are *yin* and thirty-two are *yang*. Likewise, there are thirty-two primary DNA components that, when split, create daughter cells, which become sixty-four components—which simulate the sixty-four images of the I Ching. I doubt that this is pure coincidence.

To scientists all this may be considered a discovery, but in light of ancient records it is really a rediscovery of simple basic intuitive and symbolic truths understood long before Western scientists donned their analytical hats. In the end, however, it seems the only difference lies in semantics. Quantum physics and the theories that comprise the I Ching each view life as based on thirty-two primary building blocks that have both *yin* (−) and *yang* (+) aspects. Whether these building blocks are termed as DNA or as six-lined images is irrelevant, because symbolically they mean the same thing.

It can be said that the ancient Chinese understood well that imagery is far more effective and practical to human development than is attachment to structured rationalism. Their ability of functioning in the symbolical abstract rather than in rationalism was due in part to their early association and integration of the symbolism expressed in the Eight Diagrams. Even their written language is based more on symbolism than mathematical structures of sounds, as it is in English. You need not know how to speak Chinese to read it, a unique feature not found in other languages.

The Chinese character for *I*, in fact, is a very ancient ideogram, originally meaning the chameleon, the lizard that changes its colors depending on its environment. The top portion represented the head and the four waved lines below its feet. Derived from the formation of two characters, the upper image, *jih,* refers to the "sun" or "daily," and the lower image, *wu,* represents the furling motions of banners waving. Together they give the idea of flags waving in the sunlight. Fluctuations created by the flags would cause the sunlight to change and flicker. Hence, the idea of changing light, which seemed an appropriate basis for the name for the chameleon. But the distinction in Chinese for chameleon is no longer in use, as all lizards came to be associated with dragons—the standard name for a lizard now being *shih lung tzu* (barren or stone dragon).

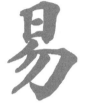

I

Sometime during the Han dynasty the character for *I* came to mean just "change," and then took on meanings like "simple," "easy," and "to treat lightly." It is very curious why the term *I* was attached to this divinational book, as it does not fit the contents of the book at all. The structure of the I Ching's text is really quite fixed. King Wen and his son, the Duke of Chou, saw to that. With all the various mandates by Heaven and the moral admonishments of the *Chuntzu* (the Wise Man), there is little room to be changeable, spontaneous, or even free willed. In brief, they laid down laws and regulations for change, which is not really spontaneous change at all. This may explain why the I Ching hit such a harmonic chord with the Confucians, and much less so with the Taoists.

Before the I Ching was put to written word and six-lined images were formed, the divination process was purely the intuition and wisdom of the diviner *(fang shih).* In the Shang dynasty, tortoise shells, bones, and bamboo slips recording various oracular readings were discovered, but no written book had been found. In this case the term *I* really fit the method.

In light of the above, there is a great deal of confusion about the diviners of ancient China. Actually, it is impossible that King Wen, the Duke of Chou, or Confucius were either experts at divination or of the diviner class *(fang shih),* because their positions would have required that they consulted with the diviners. In comparison, this would be like saying that present heads of state do all their own accounting and legal work. In present times we might say the *fang shih* class has been replaced by accountants and lawyers, for in many ways they served the same function—determining courses of action. Since it is impossible that King Wen, the Duke of Chou, or Confucius were expert diviners, why were they associated with creating a book on divination?

What is known is that divination and the theories of the I Ching existed long before the time of King Wen, as evidenced by the oracle tortoise shells and bones from the early Shang dynasty (1766–1154 B.C.E.). It is possible that King Wen converted the numerous light and dark dots of the Lo and Ho maps into solid and broken lines using yarrow stalks, rather than undergoing the cumbersome task of boring and heating of holes into tortoise shells and bones. All of this may have made the task of divination easier, and this may have something to do with the title of the classic I Ching, which can mean "easy" as well as "change." Maybe the book should be called the "Easy Book of Divination," as this certainly would have been the perception of those wanting to perform divination during those times. So if King Wen did indeed redesign the cumbersome and tedious manipulation of the dots of the Ho and Lo River Charts into the lines of the Eight Diagrams, then that was his real genius.

The actual text of the I Ching has little import for the construction of T'ai Chi postures in connection with the images, even though there are several instances where a verse does relate quite well. For example, the verse "a fox walks on thin ice" relates to the idea of how stepping occurs in T'ai Chi. Just like the fox that first tests the ice on a lake with his paw before committing his entire weight, so too the T'ai Chi practitioner must first lightly touch the heel down when stepping before committing the entire weight to the foot. Other examples appear in part 3.

The images themselves, and the *yin-yang* lines within them, however, do relate very precisely to the T'ai Chi postures. It is truly amazing how well this

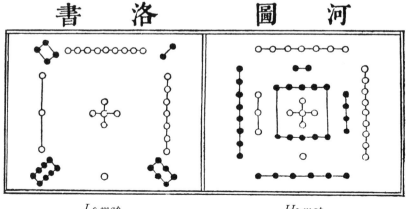

Lo map   *Ho map*

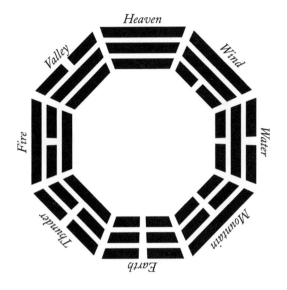

Before Heaven arrangement
of the Eight Diagrams

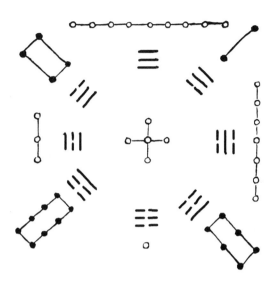

Before Heaven arrangement
correlated with the Lo map

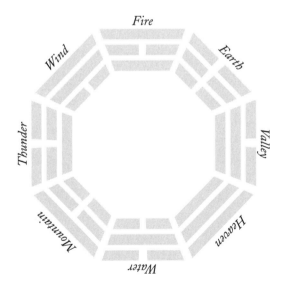

After Heaven arrangement
of the Eight Diagrams

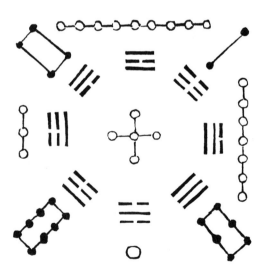

After Heaven arrangement
correlated with the Ho map

relationship of certain images to certain postures had been thought out and constructed. The images act as if they were a set of drawers, with each After Heaven, Eight Gates, and Complementary image containing a whole new facet of ideas, revealing more about a T'ai Chi posture and its functions than one could ever hope to learn from just practicing the physical movements.

Over the centuries many ways have developed in which to view the sequences and arrangements of the images of both the Eight Diagrams and the sixty-four images contained in the I Ching. In connection with the Eight Diagrams, the most common sequences are the Linear, the Square, and the Circular—shown in the Before Heaven arrangement charts in part 2 and the After Heaven charts in part 4.

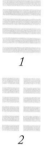

1

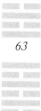

2

As for the I Ching itself, the sixty-four images are not presented in any type of systematic logic, rather in a sequence of natural change of events according to the associated names of those images. In the Ninth Wing of the I Ching (The Orderly Arrangement of the Images), each image is explained according to the influences of the previous image, the nature of the present image, and the reason for its connection with the following image. The idea is that all the images, #3 through #64, are what fill the space between Heaven (#1) and Earth (#2). The remaining sixty-two images are the events and symbolisms of what is produced between the interactions of Heaven and Earth. King Wen was most likely responsible for establishing the sequence and names for the images in the I Ching, and the logic behind this pertains more to the names of images than to the images themselves. For our purposes here, the order of the images in the I Ching serves no function.

63

64

Only in the placements of the first two images and the last two does the I Ching show any logic. The I Ching begins with the first and second images of the Creative (all solid *yang* lines) and the Receptive (all broken *yin* lines), and the last two images are #63 After Completion (Water over Fire) and #64 Before Completion (Fire over Water).

29

30

The I Ching is fashioned into two books, and Book One begins with the images of #1 The Creative (Heaven over Heaven), and #2 The Receptive (Earth over Earth). The last two images of Book One are #29 Watery Abyss (Water over Water), and #30 Illumination (Fire over Fire), not #31 and #32 as might be expected. In a loose sense of structure, however, Book One does begin with the images of Heaven over Heaven, and Earth over Earth, and ends with those of Fire over Fire, and Water over Water.

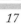

Book Two begins with #31 Concentration (Valley over Mountain) and #32 Constancy (Thunder over Wind), and the I Ching ends with #63 After Completion (Water over Fire) and #64 Before Completion (Fire over Water), which again, but even more loosely, represents the expressions and processes of the four diagonally placed images of the Eight Diagrams—Thunder, Wind, Valley, and Mountain.

The images of Thunder over Thunder, Wind over Wind, Valley over Valley, and Mountain over Mountain appear as images #17 Following, #57 Yielding, #58 Joyous, and #52 Stillness, respectively. In the end, it can be said that King Wen's arrangement of the sixty-four images has more to do with the divinational aspects of the I Ching than with any form of logic, and whatever those divinational aspects are has been lost to antiquity. I have yet to find any clear explanation for this arrangement, and even the Ninth Wing is very subjective and tenuous in its interpretation. Fortunately, the purpose of this work focuses on the *natural logic* means of interpreting the images and not the divinational, nor on the names of the images or on the structure of the sixty-four images in the I Ching.

17

57

58

52

3 Huang Ti

Teachings Attributed to the Yellow Emperor

The Yellow Emperor, Huang Ti, is the third of the Five Legendary Emperors of ancient China (Fu Hsi was the first). Huang Ti supposedly lived during China's Golden Age (2852–2255 B.C.E.) and is considered a founder of Taoism. It is reported that he spent most of his life seeking the Elixir of Immortality, and when he finally attained it, he ascended to the Immortal Realms. Although many different works are attributed to him, he cannot be seriously considered as the actual author of those various works. Through antiquity and into the present, however, his name has been chanted in praise by every Taoist. He is worshiped and revered in almost every sect of Taoism. Taoism itself was originally called "Huang Lao"—meaning someone who adhered to the teachings of Huang Ti and Lao Tzu (deemed another founder of Taoism).

The most famous of works attributed to him is the twenty-four chapter *Huang Ti Nei Ching Su Wen (Questions and Answers on the Yellow Emperor's Internal Classic),* which became the very basis of all Chinese and Japanese

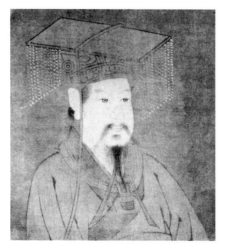

Emperor Huang Ti (the Yellow Emperor).
The third of the Five Legendary Emperors,
he supposedly ascended the throne in 2697 B.C.E.

medicine and guide for the early alchemists who sought the Elixir of Immortality. In this classic, the emperor poses various questions on health, medicine, longevity, sexual relations, and immortality to his chief minister, Ch'i Po. It is curious why this classic bears the name of Huang Ti when it is actually Ch'i Po who transmits all the knowledge.

Out of respect and veneration for his great contribution to the medical sciences, numerous medical institutions throughout China still display Huang Ti's image. In 1295, Emperor Yuan Ch'eng-tsung ordered every district of China to erect a shrine honoring Fu Hsi, Shen-Nung, and Huang Ti. Many of these shrines are reported as still intact but neglected. Surviving as the earliest and most important of all Chinese medical records, the study and applications of the *Nei Ching*, however, are still the basis for all Chinese medical students.

The *Nei Ching* has undergone countless reinterpretations and inclusions of commentaries, which is both understandable and natural for a book held in such high esteem. There is the usual problem of dating the work accurately, as with all ancient writings. Some scholars hold the view that it was without question written during the time of Huang Ti, and others say it is a Han dynasty (206 B.C.E.–22 C.E.) composition, which would place it after the appearance of the *Tao Te Ching* of Lao Tzu.

Other works attributed to the Yellow Emperor are treatises in which he converses with the divine beings *T'ien Lao (Heavenly Ancient), Su Nu (Plain Girl, a goddess of fertility), and Ts'ai Nu (Girl of Multihued Dress)*. In these manuals, Huang Ti is given instructions on the secret arts of immortality, most of which are based on transmuting the essences of male and female sexual energy in order to obtain an immortal spirit body. These works have been the basis for the Taoist practices of dual cultivation *(shuang hsiu)*, or sexual yoga *(hsing kung)*.

In present times, especially in Southeast Asia and Hong Kong, Huang Ti has become the patron immortal of divination and bringer of good fortune and protection against evil influences. Two popular booklets widely distributed in Asia show how inclusive and extensively applied the name Huang Ti has become. The first contains Taoist-Buddhist chants and a treatise titled *Huang Chih Sung Ta Hsien Chen Ching (Huang and Chih Sung's Great Immortals' True Classic)*. Chih Sung (Red Pine) was a famous Taoist immortal of the Han dynasty. The second booklet is titled *Huang Ta Hsien Ling Ch'ien (The Great Immortals' Spiritual Divination with Bamboo Slips)*.

The difficulty in interpreting the teachings of Huang Ti comes from the apparent lack of discrimination between the material and spiritual, as the view during the time of Huang Ti was that everything material contained spirit and that spirit could materialize. A good example of this is *ch'i* which not only refers to the breath but also carries the associations of vital energy, or life force, and further denotes the spirit of our emotions. *Ch'i* is associated with the weather, *t'ien ch'i,* the energy or spirit of the sky-heavens, and to *yuan ch'i,* the origin of nature's energy, which simultaneously refers to things material, spiritual, and cosmic. Numerous terms such as *ch'i* appear in the *Nei Ching,* making it difficult to determine which sense of the term (material or spiritual) is being discussed—but the dual quality of these terms also makes it easy to understand how the ancients derived their interpretations of spiritual cultivation from the classic.

In the first chapter of the *Nei Ching,* Ch'i Po's response to the first question posed by Huang Ti clearly illustrates the difficulties in interpretation. Huang Ti asks a question regarding the long life of people in ancient times before him and the negligence of people in nourishing their lives in his times. Ch'i Po answered, "People in ancient times understood the Tao (Way) and patterned their lives on the *yin* and *yang,* and so lived harmoniously with the arts of divination." Ch'i Po goes on to explain that people can live hundreds of years if they follow the natural ways of living, but because of their desires they injure their spirits and so die before their allotted time has expired.

In the quoted response of Ch'i Po, much can be interpreted about spiritual self-cultivation. The Tao is the heart of all Taoist thinking. For Ch'i Po to say the ancients understood the Tao could mean they understood the concept of Returning to the Source. To say they patterned their lives on *yin* and *yang* could mean they lived according to the natural laws and forces of nature, the ways of Heaven and Earth. To say they lived harmoniously with the arts of divination could mean that they relied on the intuitive wisdom inherent to the predictions and guidance of the spirits. The use of the term "divination" would then mean the combined sciences of astrology, the I Ching, and the calendar, all of which are regulated by the theories contained in the Supreme Ultimate (T'ai Chi), Eight Diagrams, and Five Activities.

On the other hand, Ch'i Po's answer could simply mean that the ancients lived naturally according to the ways (Tao) of men and women (*yin* and *yang*), and invoked guidance for their lives from the markings on tortoise shells and bones. We are left, and maybe rightly so, with having to decide for ourselves whether or not the implication is material or spiritual. Most likely it is both.

It is uncertain as to how the teachings of the Yellow Emperor may have influenced the later art of T'ai Chi, as there are no direct correlations between the two. The teachings on the internal development of the Immortal Spirit *(Hsien Shen),* however, would have to have had a great influence on T'ai Chi. At the very core of T'ai Chi is the goal of attaining *Shen Ming* (Illumined Spirit) and the mobilizing of *ch'i (hsing ch'i),* which are also at the core of Huang Ti's teachings. *Shen Ming* is the very state of mind the sages claimed to have sought to achieve when compiling the I Ching (see the translation of the Eighth Wing in part 2). As with the later invention of T'ai Chi, the teachings of the Yellow Emperor are motivated by the arts of self-healing, longevity, and immortality.

Within the *Nei Ching,* Ch'i Po instructs Huang Ti on what later Taoists would come to call "tortoise breathing" *(kuei hsi,* swallowing the breath), and this was the first physiological semblance of *hsing ch'i* (mobilizing the breath/*ch'i*). If the origin and date of this work is of Huang Ti and his era, then without question this would be the first written teachings on inner self-cultivation of *ch'i,* which predominates all later Taoist practices. The statement runs as follows:

> Breathe deeply seven times, each time closing up the breath *(pi ch'i),*
> extending the neck, and swallowing the breath as one does so. It should
> be as if swallowing something hard. Having done this seven times,
> move the tongue around and swallow the saliva produced several times.

T'ai Chi as we know it certainly did not exist in the time of the Yellow Emperor, but neither did Taoism as we know it. What we do know is that an emperor of antiquity is credited with much of what we now know of Taoism, from the teachings of attaining immortality, to the practice of sexual yogas, to the art of internal medicine—all so prominent in Asia. These teachings are an inherent part of T'ai Chi. The teachings attributed to this ancient emperor have influenced China and other Asian countries for nearly five thousand years. To say the Yellow Emperor did not have any influence on T'ai Chi would be remiss, and to categorically assert that he did would also be suspect, as his very person and life are in question.

4 Lao Tzu and the Tao Te Ching

The Classic on the Way and Virtue

The *Tao Te Ching* is also called the *Lao Tzu,* named after its reputed author. The name has been the object of much debate over the centuries. The character for *Lao* means "old" or "venerable" and *Tzu* can mean "son" or "master philosopher." So we can derive translations like "old son" or "the venerable philosopher(s) or master(s)." In any case, the actual existence of Lao Tzu the person is suspect and information about him is lost somewhere in China's antiquity.

What we do have is a wonderful and very popular work that has long been in China's history and has served as a main text within every sect of Taoism. In 1973 a very old copy of the *Tao Te Ching* was unearthed at Mawangtui of Changsha in Honan province, China. Buried in 168 B.C.E. (of the Later Han

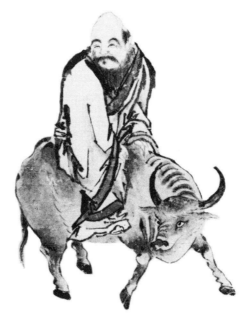

Lao Tzu riding a water buffalo

30

dynasty), this text is five centuries older than any other existing copies and its discovery has caused a great deal of debate and rethinking, as it has revealed that the teachings of Lao Tzu were present before those of Confucius. For a long time historians thought it was the other way around. Robert G. Henricks in his *Lao Tzu Te-Tao Ching* presents an excellent translation of this newly discovered text.

Lao Tzu has always been deemed, along with Huang Ti, as a founder of Taoist philosophy. Consisting of five thousand characters, his little book of eighty-one chapters is by far the most translated and printed book in the world. The history of the *Tao Te Ching*, which is quite spurious, tells us that the sage Lao Tzu decided to leave the world behind and head off to the far northwest regions of China to go into hermitage. A gatekeeper named Kuan Yin entices Lao Tzu to write a few words of instructions for posterity. Lao Tzu then wrote two short treatises, one outlining the Tao (Way) and the other *Te* (Virtue).

Within this work are wonderful aphorisms that directly relate to the very premise and heart of T'ai Chi practice. The *Tao Te Ching* at its very root is a model for leading a life void of aggression—valuing yielding over forcefulness and, most importantly, viewing virtue as the highest power of human and spiritual beings.

In regard to the practice of T'ai Chi, the most influential concept of the *Tao Te Ching* is *Wei Wu Wei*—Active Noncontention or Nonaggressive Activity. As we can surmise from its principles, T'ai Chi is completely based on this idea: *yielding* as a means of overcoming the unyielding, *learning to lose* as a means of winning without aggressive intents, *using intrinsic energy (chin)* rather than external muscular force *(li)*, and *abiding by the tan-t'ien* rather than by the reactions of the mind. The entire concept of *Wei Wu Wei* in relation to T'ai Chi can be summed up in the following two statements: "There is nothing in the world more soft and yielding than water, yet it overcomes the most hard and unyielding," and "The Tao proceeds with natural movements." Such statements have greatly influenced the principles and practices of T'ai Chi. Other examples of the philosophical relationships between T'ai Chi, the I Ching, and the *Tao Te Ching*—such as found in part 3—ultimately relate to the importance and incorporation of *Wei Wu Wei* as well.

Another very important concept Lao Tzu presented in relation to the development of T'ai Chi is found in his question, "Can you obtain the pliability of a child?" The bones of a child are soft and pliable, and the internal processes of T'ai Chi, the circulation of *ch'i,* are meant to increase and reestablish marrow to the bones, making them more pliable. A child's mind and spirit are not hindered by constraints of logic and rationalism, as implied in the Christian Bible—"have childlike faith." To have the clear and unhindered mind of a child is the ideal in Taoism. Everything in Taoism, generally speaking, relates to the idea of returning to and regenerating youthfulness, both physically and mentally. The difference is in the conscious awareness of being youthful, something the child does not have. Will Rogers's statement that "it's too bad youth is wasted on the young" seems very Taoist. The motive of T'ai Chi is identical with this Taoist thinking, to bring the body and mind back to the pliability of a child.

To live naturally in the Tao, Lao Tzu described his three treasures of humility, compassion, and frugality, which are seen in the underlying principles of T'ai Chi. No one can learn to lose, yield, or abide by the *tan-t'ien* without humility. The idea behind nonaggressive actions is compassion, as the very intent of T'ai Chi in practical use is not to injure opponents but to ward off and neutralize their aggressive actions. The idea of frugality is seen in the expedient use of movement, to use as little physical energy *(li)* as possible, relying on mind-intent *(i)* and the mobilization of *ch'i* and *shen* (spirit) to activate the motions of the body. *T'ai Chi* can then be equated, both physically and mentally, with Lao Tzu's three treasures of humility, compassion, and frugality through its principles of yielding, nonaggression, and expediency.

The relationship between T'ai Chi and the *Tao Te Ching* is purely a philosophical one, an inherent match of philosophy and physical activity—a philosophy in motion. We can see especially many correlations between the T'ai *Chi Ch'uan Treatises* and the *Tao Te Ching.* In fact, by interchanging some of its phrases, such as switching "governing the kingdom" to "regulating the body," one could easily read the *Tao Te Ching* as a *T'ai Chi Ch'uan Treatise.*

5 T'ai Chi Ch'uan Ching

The Treatises on T'ai Chi Ch'uan

Generally speaking there are three major T'ai Chi Ch'uan classical writings *(chings)* and a few dozen or so minor ones, some of which are actually parts of other writings but titled as separate treatises. These texts were revealed to the world mostly through the Chen, Yang, and Wu schools of T'ai Chi within the past one hundred years. Before Yang Lu-chan started teaching in Beijing, T'ai Chi had been hidden within strict, secret family lineages and confined to the hermitages and retreat temples of Taoist T'ai Chi practitioners.

The classical writings on T'ai Chi are infused with terms specialized for T'ai Chi and are derived from ideas and theories from many sources. Although the philosophical base of these treatises developed from the teachings of Huang Ti, the I Ching, and the *Tao Te Ching,* many other works, people, and cultural influences have appeared over the centuries to aid in T'ai Chi's formation. Some examples include the works of Hua T'o, China's greatest surgeon and inventor of the Five Animal Play health exercises; the Sung-dynasty Taoist Chen Tuan, reputed inventor of the Eight Brocades *(Pa Tuan Chin)* exercises; Ko Hung, author of the *Pao P'u Tzu,* the first practical and personal account on the search for immortality; Bodhidharma and the Shaolin Buddhist Kung Fu practices; the Chou-dynasty Taoist Chuang Tzu, who provided revolutionary writings on naturalism and spontaneity. The list could go on with many others, and would even include influences from political and historical events that played a role in T'ai Chi's development.

Even though the treatises are written in a language specialized for T'ai Chi, is is easy to apply the meanings of the verses to other matters, such as meditation, military affairs, business concerns, and so forth. Aside from interpreting them for the purposes of this book, I hope the reader will pay attention to what they have to say concerning other aspects of life.

The two men attributed with writing these treatises are Chang San-feng, a Sung-dynasty Taoist monk, and his successor, Wang Chung-yueh. Both are very enigmatic persons, as the historical details of their lives are very sparse and saturated with "Wild History." There is actually no clear-cut evidence proving that either of them practiced T'ai Chi or wrote any works on the subject—but for whatever reasons their names were attached to the treatises.

The three major treatises are as follows:

T'ai Chi Ch'uan Lun (treatise or discourse), attributed to Ancestor Chang San-feng of the Sung dynasty

T'ai Chi Ch'uan Ching (classic or canon), attributed to Taoist Immortal Wang Chung-yueh of the Ming dynasty

Shih San Shih Hsing Kung Hsin (The Mental Elucidation of the Thirteen Kinetic Postures), attributed to Taoist Immortal Wang Chung-yueh

The first of these three works is translated in its entirety, but it is the final verses on the Thirteen Postures of T'ai Chi that are of special importance to the meaning of this book.

This treatise appears to have two main divisions: the first part—running from "With every movement string . . ." to "Considered in their entirety all things have this nature"—basically gives instructions on principles of T'ai Chi. The second part—beginning with "*Chang Ch'uan* (Long Boxing) is like a long river . . ." and ending with "not merely as a means to martial skill"—is mostly correlative in content. From these lines we learn much about T'ai Chi's past and foundation. First, it states that T'ai Chi is like *Chang Ch'uan,* which is one of the early forms of boxing practiced by the Chen family. The following verses then make the definite connection with T'ai Chi and the theories of the Eight Diagrams and Five Activities, calling them the Thirteen Postures.

Last, the appended verse to the treatise tells us not only that Chang San-feng is the author but also that T'ai Chi is not just a martial art but a practice for cultivating longevity as well. Some commentators have suggested that the health and longevity aspects of T'ai Chi were not such a novel idea, as Shaolin Kung Fu monks prior to Chang proclaimed that their methods were not just for defense or martial art skills, but were also for health, inner development, and spiritual growth. In the grand scheme of things, practitioners of T'ai Chi replaced the Shaolin Kung Fu Buddhist techniques, philosophies, and associations of Shaolin Kung Fu with Taoist ones, attributing texts to Taoists such as Chang San-feng and including the ideas for health and longevity. No matter what this verse may imply, the *T'ai Chi Ch'uan Treatise* is predominately

太極拳論

一舉動周身俱要輕靈尤須貫力氣宜鼓盪神宜內斂毋使有凸凹處毋使
有斷續處其根在腳發于腿主宰于腰形于手指由腳而腿而腰總須完整
一氣向前退後乃得機得勢有不得機得勢處身便散亂其病必于腰腿求
之上下前後左右皆然凡此皆是意不在外面有上即有下有前即有後有
左即有右如意要向上即寓下意若將物掀起而加以挫之之力斯其根自
斷乃壞之速而無疑虛實宜分清楚一處自有一處虛實處處總此一虛實
周身節節貫串無令絲毫間斷耳長拳者如長江大海滔滔不絕也十三勢
者掤捋擠按採挒肘靠此八卦也進步退步右顧左盼中定此五行也掤捋
擠按即坎離震兌四正方也採挒肘靠即乾坤艮巽四斜角也進退顧盼定
即金木水火土也

T'AI CHI CH'UAN TREATISE

Attributed to Ancestor Chang San-feng,
Sung Dynasty Taoist Priest of Wu-T'ang Mountain

With every movement string all the parts together,
keeping the entire body light and nimble.

Calmly stimulate the ch'i, *with the Spirit of Vitality concentrated*
internally.

Avoid deficiency and excess, avoid projections and hollows,
avoid severance and splice.

The energy is rooted in the feet, issued through the legs, directed by the
waist, and appears in the hands and fingers.

The feet, legs, and waist must act as one unit,
so that whether Advancing or Withdrawing you will be able to obtain a
superior position and create a good opportunity.

Failure to obtain a superior position and create a good opportunity results
from the body being in a state of disorder and confusion. To correct this
disorder, adjust the waist and legs.

Likewise, upward and downward, forward and backward,
leftward and rightward—all these are to be directed by
the Mind-Intent and are not to be expressed externally.

If there is above, there must be below. If there is Advancing, there must be
Withdrawing. If there is left, there must be right.

If the initial intent is upward, you must first have a downward intent.
If you want to lift something upward, you must first have
the intent of pushing downward.

Then the root will be severed, it will be immediately and certainly toppled.
Clearly discriminate the Substantial and Insubstantial. There is an aspect of

(continued)

*Substantial and Insubstantial in every part of the body. Considered in their
entirety all things have this nature.*

*Chang Ch'uan (Long Boxing) is like a long river
or great ocean rolling on without interruption.*

*The Thirteen Postures of Warding-Off,
Rolling-Back, Pressing, Pushing, Pulling,
Splitting, Elbowing, and Shouldering
are known as the Eight Diagrams* (Pa Kua).
*Advancing, Withdrawing, Looking-Left,
Gazing-Right, and Fixed-Rooting are known
as the Five Activities* (Wu Hsing).
*Warding-Off, Rolling-Back, Pressing,
and Pushing are then* Chien, K'un, K'an, *and* Li—
*of the Four Cardinal directions.
Pulling, Splitting, Elbowing,
and Shouldering are then* Sun, Chen, T'ui,
and Ken—*of the Four Diagonal directions.
Advancing, Withdrawing, Looking-Left,
Gazing-Right, and Fixed-Rooting are then
Metal, Wood, Water, Fire, and Earth.
Joined together they become
the Thirteen Postures.*

APPENDED VERSE

This treatise has been handed down by Ancestor Chang San-feng
of Wu-T'ang Mountain so that heroes and worthy men everywhere
can lengthen their lives and attain longevity, not merely as a means
to martial skill.

about martial art, not health and spiritual development. Personally, I feel researchers have missed the mark in trying to find the origin of T'ai Chi, for it had to have developed out of and in response to the Shaolin Kung Fu styles. History records that Chang San-feng had learned the Five Animal styles of Shaolin Kung Fu during his residency in the Pao-Chi mountains.

With its appended verse and all its implications, the *T'ai Chi Ch'uan Treatise* has caused more than a century of debate, study, and intrigue within the T'ai Chi world. We must keep in mind, however, that the term T'ai Chi Ch'uan is only mentioned in the title, not within the text itself. This is a very important concern because in all the texts released during the end of the Ching dynasty and Mao's takeover, the term T'ai Chi Ch'uan is found only in two of them, and then only in the titles. It would be safe to assume that T'ai Chi Ch'uan was an invented term during this period and did not exist as a boxing art under that name until the early part of this century. The term T'ai Chi was used, but only in connection with the symbol. Keeping all this in mind, I believe it is quite obvious that T'ai Chi Ch'uan was a generic term invented to describe various earlier boxing arts, which were being coalesced into the family styles of Chen, Yang, Wu, and Li. Likewise, while all these styles were being formed, the various treatises started to appear and to be released to the public.

6 Historical Origins of T'ai Chi

Chang San-feng and Chen Wang-ting

The historical origins of T'ai Chi Ch'uan are very difficult to trace and authenticate. The earliest attributed tradition says that Chang San-feng invented T'ai Chi. It is reported that Chang was born at the end of the Sung dynasty (1247 C.E.), lived through the Yuan, and died around the age of two hundred in the Ming dynasty. He was born on Lung Ho Shan (Dragon-Tiger Mountain) in Kiangsi province, southeastern China, and during his life he went by the names Chang Tung and Chang Chun-pao. After serving as a government official, Chang sold all his property and left for Ko Hung Mountain, where the Taoist immortal KoHung (author of the famous *Pao P'u Tzu*) had resided around 300 C.E. Chang searched there for a teacher who could instruct him on the secrets of alchemy, but legend has it that he did not find a good one.

Even though he learned well the teachings of KoHung, Chang left the mountain with two young disciples. Different legends conflict about who those two disciples were. One legend says that they were two boys living on KoHung Mountain as Taoist novices who wanted to leave and seek other teachings. Another legend has it that they were two young females, claiming that Chang had learned the secret arts of Huang Ti's dual sexual cultivation, and the females were his consorts. In any case, Chang and his disciples then traveled to Mt. Pao-Chi, and there he took his common name, San-feng (Three Peaks), after the three tall mountain peaks he so admired. It is believed that while he was living there he studied the Five Animal styles of Shaolin Kung Fu Ch'uan. During the Ming dynasty, there was a great rivalry between Shaolin Kung Fu Buddhists and Wu-T'ang Taoists, most of which was politically generated by outside influences. One certain fact must be kept in mind, however: the Shaolin Kung Fu styles were considered the apex of martial arts for many centuries in China. Anyone interested in martial arts would have sought out the Shaolin Kung Fu teachings, so it is not surprising nor unlikely that Chang chose to study Shaolin Kung Fu.

After Bodhidharma's death (543 C.E.), his teachings of the *I Chin Ching (Muscle Change Classic)* and *Hsi Sui Ching (Sinew Cleansing Classic)* were devel-

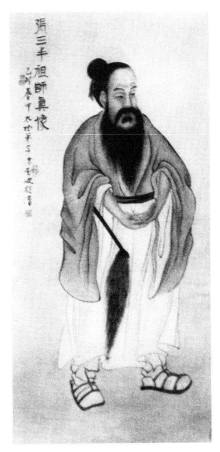

Chang San-feng, a Sung-dynasty Taoist priest
and reputed founder of T'ai Chi Ch'uan

oped into the Five Animal forms, styled after the Dragon, Tiger, Leopard, Snake, and Crane. The style that concerns our attention, however, is the Dragon. The Dragon style was based on developing lightness and agility, concentrating the spirit, complete reliance on the use of the waist and legs, and adapting to change—with the underlying premise of being in a state of tranquillity. In comparison, the Dragon style fits perfectly the description of T'ai Chi.

In Chang San-feng's biography, it is said that he became disheartened by the hardness and energy used in Shaolin Kung Fu techniques, and so he applied the Taoist theories contained in the I Ching and *Tao Te Ching* to form T'ai Chi. In the book *San Shih Erh Shih Chang Ch'uan (Thirty-Two Posture*

Long Boxing), published in 1940, the author Chin I-ming makes clear the distinction of Shaolin Kung Fu's Five Animal Ch'uan with those of Chang's Five Secret Meanings:

1. *Chin* (Intrinsic Energy) is the technique used in the Dragon style.
2. *Chin* (Adhering and Binding) is used in the Tiger style.
3. *Chin* (Approaching and Closing) is used in the Leopard style.
4. *Chi* (Attaching and Quickness) is used in the Snake style.
5. *Ch'ieh* (Severing and Effectiveness) is used in the Crane style.

So, even though it is clear that T'ai Chi developed philosophically out of Taoist and Confucian ideas, its physiological structure and history were probably more affected by Shaolin Kung Fu techniques than by any other influence. T'ai Chi certainly could not have been the product of just one man on a mountain who invented the art all on his own. It is possible, however, that Chang, from his own background in Shaolin Kung Fu techniques or from others', could have derived the methods and started the process that later developed into the art of T'ai Chi.

Chang supposedly met a Taoist hermit monk by the name of Ho Lung Hsien (Fire Dragon Immortal) who taught him the methods of achieving immortality. But after four long years of practice, he did not achieve the final goal. Along with his two disciples, Chang then went to Wu-T'ang Mountain, where after nine years of cultivating, he achieved the Tao. From then on he traveled alone, roaming different parts of China. His fame spread, and in 1385 Emperor Hsu Ti ordered him to serve as an official, but Chang ran away and hid in Yunnan province in southwest China until 1399. In 1407 Emperor Cheng Tsu then sent two officials to find him and to erect a large temple in his honor on Wu-T'ang Mountain, but again he could not be located. In 1459 Emperor Yueh Chung bestowed on him the title "The Immortal Chang." Chang, again afraid of having to serve in an official post, pretended to be mad by not bathing and by singing loudly and shouting obscene verses in public, thus he became known as "Dirty Chang."

The apocryphal legend pertaining to him is that he discovered the essence of T'ai Chi by observing a snake and magpie fighting. While sitting in his meditation hut at his mountain retreat on Wu-T'ang Mountain, Chang observed the snake being attacked by the bird. Legend claims that every time the bird would swoop down to attack the tail, the head of the snake would strike back; every time the bird attacked the head, the tail responded; and when the bird attacked the body of the snake, then both the head and tail would strike. From witnessing this event, Chang formulated the theory of T'ai Chi Ch'uan—that yielding overcomes the unyielding.

As Chang developed the movements of T'ai Chi, he achieved immortality through repeated practice of the posture "Step Back to Chase the Monkey Away." He stated that the graceful stepping back motions in combination with keeping open the *hui yin* (coccyx and perineum) aided in releasing the energy from the *hui yin* up along the spine to the top of the head. (Releasing this energy is also the reason why cross-legged sitting is always preferred in seated meditation.) It was after this event that Chang left Wu-T'ang Mountain to roam China on his own.

The debates on whether Chang San-feng actually invented T'ai Chi or not run a range of extremes. In the *Collected Records of Northern Boxing (Pei Ch'uan Hui Pien)* it states, "Chang San-feng was originally an elder disciple of Shaolin Kung Fu, and all his skills were essentially those of Shaolin Kung Fu." T'ang Tsan-sheng in his *Examination of Shaolin Kung Fu and Wu-T'ang (Shaolin Kung Fu Wu-T'ang K'ao)* responds to the above work by emphasizing that "during the time Buddhism and Taoism were first introduced and developing in China there was a huge gulf between them. How is it that a Taoist man becomes an elder disciple of Shaolin Kung Fu? A little common sense is sufficient enough to clearly distinguish the falseness in this."

The truth probably lies somewhere in between these views. On the one hand, Chang San-feng would have to have had some influences from Shaolin Kung Fu traditions—but, on the other hand, he could not have been an elder disciple of Shaolin Kung Fu. T'ang, however, makes an erroneous statement about the huge gulf between Taoism and Buddhism. A great deal of history on their long interaction disproves that notion.

In Sun Lu-t'ang's book, *The Study of T'ai Chi Ch'uan (T'ai Chi Ch'uan Hsueh),* he writes the following on Chang San-feng's invention of T'ai Chi and the correlations with the I Ching. Also within this excerpt are references to Chang's initial participation in Shaolin Kung Fu traditions:

In the time of Emperor Hsu (1333–1368 C.E.) of the Yuan dynasty, Master Chang San-feng cultivated the *Tao* in the Wu-T'ang mountains as a priest tediously cultivating the elixir, combining the training of the boxing arts (Shaolin Kung Fu) with the strengthenings of the After Heaven methods (various body strengthening exercises from the Shaolin Kung Fu traditions). But he applied these too excessively and was unable to harmonize his *ch'i*—resulting in both damaging his elixir and injuring his *yuan ch'i* (original vital energy).

Chang then decided to begin following the meanings and interpretations of two treatises, the forms of the T'ai Chi symbol and the principles of the Ho and Lo—applying the calculations of the Before Heaven of the I Ching, and put them all in accordance with the natural tendencies *(tzu jan*—"the naturally-just-so"). All of which clearly explained the mysterious and subtle methods for nourishing the body. The boxing forms and methods of the After Heaven he considered false and so there was no need to use the strengthening methods of them. Rather, he completely relied on the principles of oneness of movement, the oneness of tranquillity, and the naturally-just-so—not just on the blood and *ch'i*. He then put his full attention on Refining *Ch'i (Lien Ch'i)* and Transforming Spirit *(Hua Shen)*, which were all contained within the mysterious and profound meanings of the One Principle *(I Li)*, Two Powers *(Liang I)*, Three Powers *(San Tsai)*, Four Emblems *(Szu Hsiang)*, Five Activities *(Wu Hsing)*, Six Unions *(Lui Ho)*, Seven Star *(Ch'i Hsing)*, Eight Diagrams *(Pa Kua)*, and Nine Palaces *(Chiu Kung)*.

In the beginning there is the One, in the end, the Nine. The calculations of the Nine likewise revert back to the One.

The **One Principle** means: the beginning point of the art of T'ai Chi Ch'uan dwells in the harmonizing of the *ch'i* within the abdomen—this is T'ai Chi.

The **Two Powers** means: the application of oneness of movement and the oneness of tranquillity of the entire body—this is *Liang I* (the Two Powers of *yin* and *yang)*.

The **Three Powers *(San Tsai)*** means: the head, hands, and feet; and the upper, middle, and lower parts of the body.

The **Four Emblems *(Szu Hsiang)*** means: advancing to the front, withdrawing to the back, looking to the left, and gazing to the right.

The **Five Activities *(Wu Hsing)*** means: Advancing, Withdrawing, Looking-Left, Gazing-Right, and Fixed-Rooting.

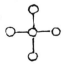

The ***Six Unions (Lui Ho)*** means: uniting the *shen* (spirit) with the *ching* (regenerative energy), uniting the *ch'i* with the *shen*, and uniting the *ching* with the *ch'i*—these are the three Internal Unions. Uniting the shoulders with the hips, uniting the elbows with the knees, and uniting the hands and feet—these are the three External Unions. Internally and externally these are in essence the same, and they complete the Six Unions.

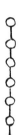

The ***Seven Stars (Ch'i Hsing)*** means: the head, hands, shoulders, elbows, hips, knees, and the feet, which are also called the Seven Fists *(Ch'i Ch'uan)*—these are the Seven Stars.

The ***Eight Diagrams (Pa Kua)*** means: Warding-Off, Rolling-Back, Pressing, Pushing, Pulling, Splitting, Elbowing, and Shouldering—these are the Eight Diagrams.

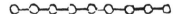

The ***Nine Palaces (Chiu Kung)*** means: the Eight Hands *(Pa Shou)* in conjunction with the Central Fixed Position *(Chung Ting)*, which are all connected with the Eight Diagrams.

The master taking the treatises of the Ho map and Lo River Charts, the Appendixes *(Ten Wings of the I Ching)*, the Eight Diagrams and Nine Palaces, the Five Activities, and the applications of the Seven Stars and Eight Diagrams thereby created the art of T'ai Chi Ch'uan.

During his years of roaming, Chang San-feng's disciple, Wang Tsung, reportedly taught Chen Tung-chou, who taught Chang Sung-hsi (from Hai-yen of Chekiang province) during the mid-1500s. Chang then taught Yeh Chi-ma, who taught Wang Chung-yueh, a native of Tai Hang Mountains in Shansi province. Wang then taught Chiang Fa, a native of Hobei province, who then taught Chen Wang-ting of the Chen family, native of Honan province. Assuming Chang San-feng as the founder, this is the most logical lineage leading up to Chen Wang-ting—although other traditions differ.

The difficulty in verifying Chang San-feng as the founding teacher is that many Taoist monks during this period used the same surname of Chang, taken from the lineages of Chang Tao-ling, the first Taoist pope. But none of these Changs could be directly associated with T'ai Chi Ch'uan, and neither can Chang San-feng himself.

In *Self and Society in Ming Thought*, the author Anna Seidel provides an excellent and well-researched piece on Chang San-feng in the chapter "A Taoist Immortal of the Ming Dynasty: Chang San-feng." Seidel presents a great deal of evidence proving his existence during the Ming dynasty, but she could not prove his association with T'ai Chi. So it is still uncertain as to whether or not his invention of T'ai Chi is a fabrication of later T'ai Chi masters.

Chang supposedly left behind another treatise, *Chang San-feng's T'ai Chi Lien Tan Mi Shou (Chang San-feng's Secret Explanations on T'ai Chi and Refining the Elixir of Immortality)*, but it is doubtful that he is the original author. It is from this treatise that I drew the majority of the legends about him.

Although it is more likely that Wang Chung-yueh's disciple, Chiang Fa, actually taught Chen Wang-ting, another tradition claims that it was actually Wang who had done so. Supposedly while wandering in Honan province, Wang came across Chen Wang-ting's family, who were practicing boxing arts called *Pao Ch'uan* (Cannon Fist) and *Chang Ch'uan* (Long Boxing). After defeating the better skilled members of the family, Wang decided to stay and teach the Chens the deeper aspects of his boxing art, called *Nei Ch'uan* (Inner Boxing), which the Chens had to have considered as far superior to their old styles. Wang modified their boxing style and the assumption is that the Chens later called these methods T'ai Chi. This story may explain the two seemingly distinct systems within the Chen family tradition of Old Style and New Style.

For five generations afterward, the Chens produced great T'ai Chi masters and incorporated many changes since the founder Chen Wang-ting's time. The Chen family is still in place at Chen Family Village in Honan province, and the Chinese government considers them a national treasure.

The most profound development in T'ai Chi's history, however, occurred during the early 1800s when Yang Lu-chan (1799–1872) learned the boxing arts from the Chen family. Posing initially as a deaf mute to acquire a servant's job, Yang Lu-chan secretly learned T'ai Chi at Chen Family Village (Chen Chia Kuo) in Hopei province. Spying on their practice sessions, he learned much of their art, and after thirteen years he left and went to Beijing to teach publicly, the first T'ai Chi master to do so. His Yang Family Style was much different from the Chen Style, and his open manner of teaching soon became very popular with the masses—and has continued to be so into present times.

Another tradition, and more believable, says that Yang was purchased as a servant boy along with his friend, Li Po-kuei, in a drugstore owned by one of the Chens and was taught T'ai Chi because he was then considered as a part of the family. In any event, his skills became so good that he defeated all the students within the Chen family, and the head of the family at that time, Chen Ch'ang-hsin, took personal interest in him and taught him as much as he could about T'ai Chi.

When Yang decided to leave Chen Family Village, the family honored him with a banquet and money. (When he died in 1872, his body was returned and buried at Chen Family Village, a very high and unheard of honor within Chinese family traditions. Yang's headstone still remains outside the main gate at Chen Family Village.)

Yang went back to his home in Yung Lien Hsien in Hopei and landed jobs working in a drugstore and teaching T'ai Chi. The store owner, Wu Yu-hsiang, was also interested in boxing, and he and Yang became close friends. Because of his friendship with Yang, Wu also decided to go and learn from the Chens. It is reported that during his month-long stay there he acquired T'ai Chi documents attributed to Wang Chung-yueh. After returning he shared these notes with Yang and Wu's two brothers, Wu Ju-ching and Wu Ch'iu-ying. Both of Wu's brothers were men of letters, and Ju-ching later wrote five papers on T'ai Chi.

Yang and Wu Ju-ching later went to Beijing to teach T'ai Chi, and Yang acquired many students. It was there that Yang acquired the title "Yang the Unbeatable"—a testament to his proficiency in the art of boxing. It was also during this time that the *T'ai Chi Ch'uan Treatise* attributed to Chang San-feng was most likely compiled. In this classic, the verse "*Chang Ch'uan* (Long Boxing) is like a long river or great ocean flowing on without interruption" is of particular interest, as *Chang Ch'uan* was the name of a style of boxing that the Chens had practiced since the time of Chen Wang-ting, and curiously enough was in the title of the treatise that Wu Yu-hsiang had acquired from the Chens—*Thirteen Postures of Long Boxing* by Wang Chung-yueh.

Backtracking a bit here, it is also claimed that the Taoist Chang Sung-hsi, the third disciple mentioned above in the Chang San-feng lineage, was a learned scholar who had a special interest in the I Ching—as did most Taoist adepts. If this claim is true then it would be very possible that he would have been the initial source of matching the workings of T'ai Chi and the I Ching together, which then suggests that he handed down these ideas to Yeh

Chi-ma, who passed them to Wang Chung-yueh, who passed them to Chiang Fa, who in turn gave copies to Chen Wang-ting. Chang Sung-hsi's ideas could then have been part of the documents Wu Yu-hsiang had acquired from the Chens, which would explain how all these ideas were passed on through Yang Lu-chan and his disciples and why the treatises attributed to Chang San-feng started surfacing in public.

In 1957 a book was published in Taipei—*Wang Tsung Hsien Sheng Nan Chuan T'ai Chi Ch'uan (Master Wang Tsung's Southern History of T'ai Chi Ch'uan)* by Ni Ching-ho—that gave credence to the belief in Chang San-feng and his lineage passing down to Wang Chung-yueh. This work presents several treatises attributed to Wang Tsung, Chen Tung-chou, Wang Chung-yueh, and Chang San-feng. Ni claims lineage from Huang Li-chou, author of the *Nanlei Anthology,* who claims to have practiced and learned the boxing art *Nei Ch'uan* from Wang Chung-yueh.

It was Huang Li-chou in the Ming dynasty who first associated Chang San-feng with being the founder of T'ai Chi and listed the lineages to Wang Chung-yueh. Yang's students, among whom there were a few scholars, including Wu Yu-hsiang and his two brothers Ch'iu-ying and Ju-ching, and Chen Wei-ming, all could easily have read Huang's work and used it as the basis for placing Chang San-feng as the founder of T'ai Chi. One could then assume that they added the references of *Chang Ch'uan, Pa Kua,* and *Wu Hsing* to the *T'ai Chi Ch'uan Treatise,* which established T'ai Chi's association to the I Ching.

It was also during these years of China's upheaval, the Boxer Rebellion, the Opium Wars, and the fall of the Ching dynasty, that not only T'ai Chi took form, but Pa Kua Chang (Eight Diagram Palms) and Hsing-I Ch'uan (Intent Form Boxing) were also coming into their own. Pa Kua Chang was developed entirely on the theories of the Eight Diagrams, Hsing-I Ch'uan through the Five Activities, and both gradually became known as sister arts of T'ai Chi.

In conclusion, it is safe to assume that during the final years of the Ming dynasty, Chen Wang-ting and other members of his family learned T'ai Chi from Wang Chung-yueh or Chiang Fa and other boxers. Later, in the early 1800s of the Ching dynasty, Yang Lu-chan learned these boxing skills from the Chens. Yang then taught Wu Yu-hsiang and his two brothers Ch'iu-yin, and Ju-ching and their cousin Li I-yu. Yang and Wu Ju-ching went to teach T'ai Chi in Beijing in possession of various T'ai Chi documents secured by

Wu Yu-hsiang. Yang and Ju-ching must then have assigned one of those treatises to Chang San-feng, which probably originated from Huang Li-chou's early claim.

That Yang and Ju-ching possessed information suggesting Chang San-feng was the founder of T'ai Chi is believable and probable. That they would attribute the treatise to Chang San-feng also suggests that they attached the concluding and appended verses to the treatise as well. This would make sense if we accept that they possessed the information that linked T'ai Chi to I Ching philosophy—and that they were simply passing on information they had acquired.

PART II

The Framework of I Ching T'ai Chi

7 The T'ai Chi Symbol

(T'ai Chi T'u)

The T'ai Chi symbol is a dialectical representation of *yin* and *yang*, male and female, light and dark, being and nonbeing, negative and positive, Heaven and Earth—in essence, it is a symbolic expression of the interplay and constantly changing aspects of all dualistic aspects inherent in our world and universe.

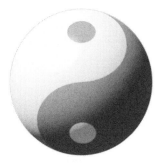

The term T'ai Chi is associated with both its philosophical representation, as shown in the double-fish symbol, and as an abbreviated name for T'ai Chi Ch'uan. Properly, T'ai Chi should be used only in reference to the double-fish symbol and its associated philosophy. The movements of T'ai Chi Ch'uan should include the term Ch'uan (boxing or fists). The abbreviated "T'ai Chi," however, has become such an accepted term for the movements that I have chosen to maintain its usage. Consequently, when speaking of the T'ai Chi image in this chapter, I attach the word "symbol" or "image" to it, and/or italicize it, so as to avoid any confusion.

The origination of the term T'ai Chi in conjunction with the use of the T'ai Chi symbol is buried somewhere in China's antiquity. Evidence suggests that it was associated with the early shamans and divinators, and in early Taoist philosophy, the meaning of T'ai Chi, both as a term and symbol, developed out of stories from much earlier concepts of the Cosmic Egg and the legends of Pan Ku, the mythical creator of the universe. An egg is much like the T'ai Chi symbol, with its insides containing the egg white and the yoke, representing the *yin* and *yang* aspects of all things. Another view holds that since early humans were completely at the mercy of and dependent upon nature's forces, nature's dialectical opposites—such as the opposite effects of Heaven and Earth (sky and soil), male and female (reproduction)—would have been more than apparent to them. It was then very natural for them to perceive things in terms of *yin* and *yang*—which originated from calling the sunny, south side of a mountain *yang,* and the shaded, north side *yin.*

In the forty-second chapter of the *Tao Te Ching,* Lao Tzu writes, "Tao produced the One, the One produced Two, Two produced Three, Three produced the Ten-Thousand Things." This was taken later to mean Tao produced the T'ai Chi (One), T'ai Chi produced *Yin* and *Yang* (Two), *Yin* and *Yang* produced Three (*San Tsai*—Heaven, Earth, and Man), and *San Tsai* produced *Wan Wu* (the Ten-Thousand Things).

Chuang Tzu used the terms *T'ai I* (Grand Unity) and *Ta I* (The Great Oneness). But like Lao Tzu, their references are not specific enough to determine concretely that the T'ai Chi symbol was their invention or model.

The confusion has always been that the original concept of the T'ai Chi symbol was that it antedated creation, and later came to represent the *yin* and *yang* influences that unified or reconciled creation. The idea of dual forces governing creation date so far back into Chinese history that it is difficult to speculate anything concerning its origin. Ideas like the Hun and P'o spirits (Heavenly and Earthly souls uniting to form a human life), the Gourd (representing being and nonbeing), and the Cosmic Egg all share a common bond with the philosophic concept of the T'ai Chi symbol.

The T'ai Chi symbol has undergone many changes through the course of its history and development. We see it as a symbol of two fish; male and female, interlocking in reproduction; as white and dark concentric half circles integrating with each other; and in a variety of other depictions. They all carry the same meaning and all developed from the theories of the changing *yin* and *yang* lines.

In many publications the T'ai Chi symbol is positioned incorrectly. The proper position of this image (as shown on page 51) is with the large white area positioned on the top left, and the large dark portion on the bottom right. This is so Heaven maintains a *yang,* southerly position, and Earth a *yin,* northerly position.

The clarification of the T'ai Chi symbol came during the period of eleventh-century Confucianism from two famous neo-Confucian Sung-dynasty scholars, Chou Tun-i (1017–1073) and Chu Hsi (1130–1200), who used it to represent the Absolute or the Illimitable. Chou Tun-i wrote two short treatises explaining the theories of the philosophy of T'ai Chi—*T'ai Chi T'u Shou (Treatise on the Symbolism of the Supreme Ultimate)* and *T'ung Shu (Penetrating the I Ching)*. Because of his work, I think it is justified to say that Chou Tun-i invented the T'ai Chi symbol and its philosophy as we know it today. Chu Hsi basically took Chou Tun-i's works and built on them, and is credited with explaining the nature of T'ai Chi, something Chou did not do. It is interesting that a philosophical concept that was largely developed by Confucians has become the symbol most associated with Taoism and not neo-Confucianism.

Chou Tun-i's *Treatise on the Symbolism of the Supreme Ultimate* fully describes the meaning of the T'ai Chi symbol, and it is presented here in its entirety.

TREATISE ON THE SYMBOLISM OF THE SUPREME ULTIMATE

by Chou Tun-i

WU CHI (THE ULTIMATE OF NONBEING) AND T'AI CHI (THE SUPREME ULTIMATE OF BEING)

Through movement the Supreme Ultimate produces *yang*. When movement reaches its limit, it becomes tranquil. Through tranquillity the Supreme Ultimate produces *yin*. When tranquillity reaches its limit, movement begins again. Movement and tranquillity alternate and are the source of each other. From them are born the distinctions of *yin* and *yang*, and the two operations are firmly established.

From the transformations of *yang* and its union with *yin*, the Five Attributes *(Wu Hsing)* of Water, Fire, Wood, Metal, and Earth manifest. When these five *ch'i* (energies or forces) are orderly and harmoniously distributed, the Four Seasons run their natural course.

The Five Attributes represent one system of *yin* and *yang*, and *yin* and *yang* represent one Supreme Ultimate. The Supreme Ultimate (T'ai Chi) is fundamentally the Ultimate of Nonbeing *(Wu Chi)*, and the Five Activities come from these, and each contain their specialized natures.

When *Wu Chi* and the essences of *yin-yang* and the Five Attributes mysteriously unite, integration occurs. Chien (Heaven) represents the male activity, and K'un (Earth) represents the female activity. The intercourse of these two material forces generates and transforms all things (Wan Wu). All things produce and reproduce, creating an unending process of transformations.

Man alone acquires the highest excellences of the Five Attributes and is therefore the most intelligent of all things. From them his physical form appears, and his spirit develops consciousness. Because of this consciousness the Five Moral Principles arise and he then engages in activity, creating reactions to the external world. From this activity good and evil are distinguished, and human affairs come about.

It is the sage *(sheng jen)* who can discern these affairs through the principles of the Mean, Correctness, Humanity, and Virtuousness— the way of the sage constitutes these four principles. The sage regards tranquillity as fundamental—without desire there will be tranquillity. Through tranquillity the sage establishes himself as the ultimate example of Man. The nature of the sage is identical with Heaven and Earth; his brilliance is identical with the sun and moon; his orderly conduct is identical with the Four Seasons; and his good fortunes and misfortunes are identical with those of the spiritual beings *(kuei shen)*. The superior man cultivates these moral attributes and benefits from good fortune, but the inferior man violates them and experiences misfortune.

Therefore, it is said, *"Yin* and *yang* are the Way (Tao) of Heaven, the weak and strong the Way of Earth, and humanity and virtue the Way of Man." It is also said, "Investigating the cyclic changes of phenomena, we will understand the concept of life and death." Great is the I Ching and its excellence!

In this treatise Chou created a type of chronological order of the production of material forces. First there is *Wu Chi* and then the *T'ai Chi*. Because of movement, *yang* appears, and when it reaches its extreme, *yin* appears. When *yin* reaches its extreme, *yang* appears again—a never-ending cycle of change. These cycles of change between *yin* and *yang* produce the Five Attributes, each of which has a *yin* and *yang* aspect to it, and from them the Four Seasons develop. With them, *Chien* and *K'un* come about, creating *Wan Wu* (all things, or the Ten-Thousand Things) and the unending cycle of life and death, production and reproduction. We must note that Chou places the production of the Five Attributes before that of the Eight Diagrams, which was the fashion of Confucian thinking in his day. Later, Taoists switched the order, listing the Eight Diagrams as creating the Five Attributes.

Chu Hsi clarified much of Chou's treatise in his work *The Supreme Ultimate* using very polite arguments about what T'ai Chi is. He first extended the meaning of material forces to include the concept that they must have principle *(li)*, which is a verification of Confucian ideals. Chou hints at this idea when he says, "The Five Attributes are seen in man through the Five Moral Principles," but Chu Hsi extends this meaning to everything—Tao, Heaven and Earth, *yin* and *yang,* Four Seasons, and all things *(Wan Wu).*

Chu Hsi becomes more Taoist in approach when commenting on what the T'ai Chi is and its function. Some of his more important remarks are as follows:

> T'ai Chi is not something that exists in chaos before the creation of Heaven and Earth but is a generic term for the principles of Heaven and Earth and all things.
>
> Within all things there is the T'ai Chi. Fundamentally, there is only one T'ai Chi, but like the one moon, its light casts upon all the rivers and lakes. We cannot say the moon divides itself to accomplish this.
>
> The T'ai Chi is bound neither by space nor physical form. It has no fixed place or position.
>
> *Yin* and *yang* only exist after physical form is part of them. Movement is, after all, the motion *(yang)* of T'ai Chi, as tranquillity is the tranquilness *(yin)* of T'ai Chi, even though movement and tranquillity are not in themselves T'ai Chi.
>
> After the occurrence of activity, T'ai Chi results. Changing to tranquillity, it still exists, unending.
>
> All of this is vague, but the truth of T'ai Chi must be personally realized by each and every one of us.

The last statement of Chu Hsi echoes clearly the words of Lao Tzu, "The Tao that can be Tao'ed is not the eternal Tao. The name that can be named is not the everlasting name." All philosophies that try to explain the source of things are inevitably confounded by the use of words. Chu Hsi is correct in ending his discussion by advising that we must experience this truth for ourselves, not through the words and explanations of others.

Toward the end of the Ming dynasty, we come to the materials attributed to Wang Chung-yueh. In his treatise *T'ai Chi Ch'uan Ching,* his opening verse runs, "T'ai Chi is born of *Wu Chi,* the mother of *yin* and *yang.* In motion they separate, in tranquillity they unite."

Later he states, *"Yin* is not separate from *yang,* and *yang* is not separate from *yin."* This statement is unquestionably derived from the works of Chou Tun-i and Chu Hsi.

In Tung Ying-chieh's book *T'ai Chi Ch'uan Shih I (The Principles and Meanings of T'ai Chi Ch'uan),* published in 1948, a minor treatise, *The T'ai Chi Circle,* expounds well the use of the waist in T'ai Chi, which is the body's symbolic representation of the T'ai Chi symbol.

THE T'AI CHI CIRCLE

Withdrawing and circling is easy, but Advancing and circling is the most difficult.

Never separate the waist and the top of the head, or back and front, as it will then be difficult to keep separating from your center-Earth position.

Withdrawing is easy, Advancing is difficult. You must study them carefully. This statement refers to the skills of movement, and not to standing in equilibrium.

When seeking to take advantage of the opponent's body with Advancing and Withdrawing, the shoulders must unite together; just like a water-mill tread, churning fast and slow, or like a dragon in the clouds or a tiger in the wind, the image is that of roundness and circling.

By applying the Circle of Heaven to seek the goal, everything will eventually come about and happen naturally.

8 Fu Hsi's Before Heaven Arrangement of the Eight Diagrams

As stated earlier, during China's Golden Age, the Five Legendary Emperors (approximately 3000 B.C.E.), history reports of a mythical sage-ruler named Fu Hsi. As the first emperor of China, Fu Hsi is credited with having invented the *Pa Kua,* or Eight Diagrams—which eventually led to the formation of the I Ching, the sixty-four images. The graphic below shows Fu Hsi's arrangement of the Eight Diagrams, and the subsequent paragraphs describe two manners in which this arrangement can be read, showing how the images relate and transform into each other.

We can see that from the topmost image, Heaven (three *yang,* or solid, lines), and moving down along the left side of the arrangement to Valley (one *yin,* or broken, line, and two *yang* lines), the topmost line has changed to *yin.* Next, in

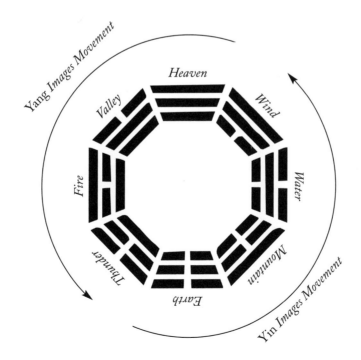

Fire (one *yang,* one *yin,* and a *yang* line), the second line changed to *yin.* Lastly, in Thunder (two *yin* and one *yang* line), both the top and middle lines changed to *yin.* This completes the changes of the *yang* images.

In the second phase of the *yin* images, the changes occur moving upward along the right side of the arrangement. First, the bottom image of Earth (three *yin* lines) changes into Mountain (two *yin* and one *yang* line)—in which the topmost line changed to *yang.* Mountain then changes to Water (one *yin,* one *yang,* and one *yin* line), in which the second line changed to *yang.* Lastly, in Wind (two *yang* and one *yin* line), both the top and middle lines changed to *yang.* At this point, because *yin* has reached its extreme it will change into *yang* again, Heaven.

Yang *Images:*

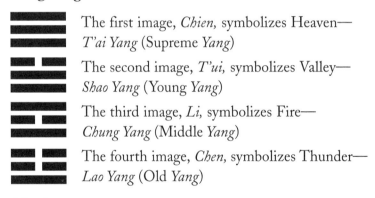

The first image, *Chien,* symbolizes Heaven—
T'ai Yang (Supreme *Yang*)

The second image, *T'ui,* symbolizes Valley—
Shao Yang (Young *Yang*)

The third image, *Li,* symbolizes Fire—
Chung Yang (Middle *Yang*)

The fourth image, *Chen,* symbolizes Thunder—
Lao Yang (Old *Yang*)

Yin *Images:*

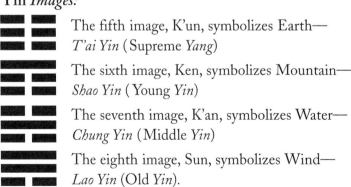

The fifth image, K'un, symbolizes Earth—
T'ai Yin (Supreme *Yang*)

The sixth image, Ken, symbolizes Mountain—
Shao Yin (Young *Yin*)

The seventh image, K'an, symbolizes Water—
Chung Yin (Middle *Yin*)

The eighth image, Sun, symbolizes Wind—
Lao Yin (Old *Yin*).

Another manner in which to view these images is to proceed the same as before, from Heaven down to Thunder, but to then move to Thunder's opposite, or complementary, image of Wind, and proceed downward on the right side of the arrangement to Earth.

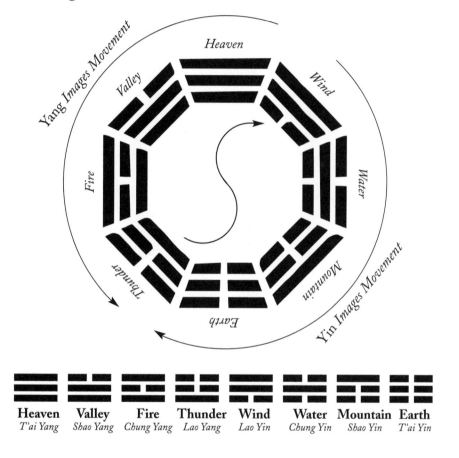

Heaven	Valley	Fire	Thunder	Wind	Water	Mountain	Earth
T'ai Yang	*Shao Yang*	*Chung Yang*	*Lao Yang*	*Lao Yin*	*Chung Yin*	*Shao Yin*	*T'ai Yin*

These Eight Diagrams symbolize all the phenomena in our world and are known collectively as the Before Heaven images. These images are formed from combining single *yang* (solid) and *yin* (broken) lines. Each image contains three lines, culminating in eight separate images, totaling twenty-four lines. These numbers are extremely important, as the three lines represent the idea of Heaven, Earth, and Man (discussed later). The eight images, comprised of four *yang* diagrams and four *yin* diagrams, represent the four basic elements of creation (Heaven, Earth, Fire, and Water) and the four expressions of creation (Wind, Thunder, Valley, and Mountain), as well as the eight phases of the moon and the eight directions. The twenty-four lines, twelve *yin* and twelve *yang*, represent not only the twenty-four divisions of the Chinese calendar year, but time as well. The Chinese measurement of daily time is divided into twelve, two-hour periods, with each period being further divided into both a *yin* and *yang* hour. All of these images, numbers, and representations can be applied to any aspect associated within the workings of Heaven, Earth, or Man. Thus, by extension, they form a complete imagery representation of our phenomenal world.

In the earliest records the images of Fire *(Li)* and Water *(K'an)* were associated more specifically with Sun (Fire) and Moon (Water). The imagery of Heaven, Earth, Sun, and Moon were then seen as representing the four primary positions of the arrangement, and Mountain, Valley, Thunder, and Wind represented the four minor positions of the arrangement.

It can only be speculated as to why the terms Fire and Water were ultimately exchanged for Sun and Moon. The most logical assumption is that Confucian scholars rejected using Sun and Moon because these terms were found within Taoist sexual alchemy practices, which moralist Confucians would not accept. Taoism then cloaked their sexual symbolisms with terms like "red (fire/male) and white (water/female)" and "dragon (sun/male) and tiger (female/ water)."

The use of Fire and Water do represent *Li* and *K'an* well, however, as the sun is the ultimate expression of Fire, and the moon is the ultimate influence on the tides of the oceans, seas, and thus all bodies of water on the Earth. Fire and Water have been the standard terms used for the images of *Li* and *K'an* since the Chou dynasty.

The Before Heaven arrangement of the Eight Diagrams, in connection with the T'ai Chi symbol, has three manners for moving through the images: (1) moving from one complementary image to another—such as Heaven to Earth, Valley to Mountain, and so on; (2) moving counterclockwise from Heaven around the circle; and (3) moving from Heaven down to Thunder, then across to Wind and then down to Earth.

1. Moving through the complements of the T'ai Chi symbol

The Eight Diagrams, like the sixty-four hexagrams of the I Ching, are also arranged to depict our world's complementary dual functions and pairing of opposites.

Heaven and **Earth**

Valley and **Mountain**

Fire and **Water**

Thunder and **Wind**

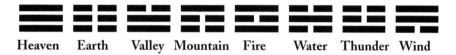

Heaven **Earth** **Valley** **Mountain** **Fire** **Water** **Thunder** **Wind**

This pairing of opposites is how the *T'ai Chi Ch'uan Treatise* likewise arranges the Eight Postures of T'ai Chi—which is the standard by which the 16-Posture I Ching T'ai Chi Form was constructed.

2. Moving around the T'ai Chi symbol

In the Before Heaven arrangement, the *yang* movement of the images goes to the left and down, and the *yin* movements run to the right and up. Hence, the three *yang* lines of Heaven gradually descend to just one *yang* line (Thunder), as the number of *yin* lines increases. Likewise, the three *yin* lines of Earth gradually ascend to just one *yin* line (Wind), as the number of *yang* lines now increases. So in reaching Wind, with its two *yang* lines, the number of *yang* lines increases to three and we are back at Heaven again. Just as is seen on the other end of the spectrum, as the number of *yang* lines decreases and the number of *yin* lines increase, the two *yin* lines of Thunder then transform into the three *yin* lines of Earth.

The descriptions of the movements of *yin* and *yang* need some clarification here, as the *yin* aspect of movement sounds strange at first—meaning, how can *yin* ascend from three lines (Earth) to one line (Wind)? This can be explained within the nature of *yin* itself, which naturally moves downward. *Yang* is light, so it naturally causes things to rise, while *yin* is heavy and causes things to sink. Because Heaven has reached its fullest point of *yang* energy—three *yang* lines—it can then only start to become *yin* and must decrease in strength. This decrease in strength, however, means that *yin* is increasing in strength. So the downward movement and decline of *yang* energy is naturally increasing *yin*'s strength. But when *yin* is decreasing in strength, its energy must then ascend. Therefore, Earth, with its three *yin* lines, ascends to Wind, with its one *yin* line.

In summary, this manner of moving through the images can be seen as tracing the energy of either the *yang* or *yin* movement. So in starting with Heaven, the *yang* energy descends from its strongest point of three *yang* lines to no *yang* lines (Earth), and then increases in strength and ascends to Heaven again. If we examine the movement from the *yin* point of view, also starting with the image for Heaven, the *yin* energy moves downward from no *yin* lines, but increases to its fullest strength of three *yin* lines when it reaches the bottom, the position for Earth. Then as the images ascend back to Heaven, *yin* loses its strength, moving from three *yin* lines to no *yin* lines as the movement goes full circle to Heaven.

3. Moving through the T'ai Chi symbol

As in the second manner, at first there is a descending movement of the images to the left and down, from Heaven to Valley to Fire to Thunder—but from here Thunder transforms into Wind (following the natural curve of the T'ai Chi symbol). The movement continues descending on the right and down, from Wind to Water to Mountain and to Earth. This pattern of movement starts from the position of Heaven and describes how the *yang* energy decreases and starts moving left and down. The difference here is that it continues to show the downward descent of *yang* through the other images as well, until reaching Earth, where the *yang* energy is at its weakest. This pattern of movement, on the other hand, is tracing the increase of *yin* energy through all the images as well.

These three manners for examining the Before Heaven arrangement of the Eight Diagrams are very basic, and the theories and correlations stemming from them are much more involved than what has been presented here. However, these brief descriptions serve well as a background for the later associations with the construction of the T'ai Chi postures.

In the *Ten Wings of the I Ching*, the Eighth Wing, *Treatise on the Diagrams (Shou Kua Ch'uan)*, provides a broad list of associations for each diagram. The treatise actually contains eleven sections, but as an introduction I present the first three. The remaining eight sections are but correlations of the images, and most of these I compiled into the Eight Diagrams Correlation Chart, which follows the treatise.

TREATISE ON THE EIGHT DIAGRAMS
The Eighth Wing of the I Ching
by Confucius (Kung Fu Tzu)

Section One

In ancient times, when the sages were compiling the I Ching, they sought mysterious assistance for their spiritual wisdom *(Shen Ming)*, and so created the regulations for using the divining plant (yarrow stalks or the milfoil plant).

The number three was assigned to Heaven, and the number two to Earth, and from these the calculation of all the other numbers came.

The sages contemplated the changes in the divided *(yin)* and undivided *(yang)* lines by using the stalks, and formed images *(Pa Kua)*. From the movements that occur between the strong *(yang)* and weak *(yin)* lines, they were then able to assemble their teachings on each of the separate lines. There was then produced a harmonious conformity with that of the Way (Tao) and Virtue *(Te)*, to aid in the decision of what was right for each image. They made exhaustive discriminations of these rightnesses, with the effect that the nature of each of them was completely developed, and arrived at the decree of Heaven's appointment.

Section Two

Formerly, when the ancients compiled the I Ching, it was designed so that the images would be in conformity with both the principles of the basic natures of humankind and all things, and with the regulations appointed for them by Heaven. In doing this, they revealed the Way of Heaven by calling the lines *yin* and *yang*, the Way of Earth by calling the lines *weak* and *strong*, the Way of Man by calling the lines *benevolence* and *righteousness*. Each image [trigram] then embraces the Three Powers. With the images stacked upon each other, there were then six lines in the full image [hexagram]. The distinctions [Three Powers] were assigned with either *yin* or *yang* lines, occupying their proper positions within the images [hexagrams] so that each of the images was completed.

Section Three
The images of Heaven and Earth received their fixed positions. Mountains and Valleys were to interchange their influences on each other. Thunder and Wind were to create excitement to the other. Water and Fire were to do each other no injury. In this way there was mutual communication between all the Eight Images.

Calculating the past is natural logic and acquiring knowledge of the future is forecasting. Therefore, in the I Ching there is both natural logic and forecasting.

In the Chinese way of thinking, nothing has much worth unless it can be applied to either or both the *Pa Kua* (Eight Images or Diagrams) and *Wu Hsing* (the Five Elements, Agents, or Activities) theories. They are the very fabric on which T'ai Chi is based. In fact, T'ai Chi was originally called "Thirteen Posture Boxing" for the very reason of its integration of the *Pa Kua* and *Wu Hsing* theories.

The Before Heaven *(Fu Hsi)* arrangement represents what we might call the internal expressions of phenomena in the world. The After Heaven (King Wen) arrangement then reveals what is in the external world. Heaven (*yang*, male, and sun), Earth (*yin*, female, and moon), Water (blood and nourishment), Fire (*ch'i* and warmth), Valley (abdomen and emptiness), Wind (breath and movement), Thunder (sinews and reactions), Mountain (bones and stillness)—these types of dialectics can be expanded to greater and greater distinctions, and I encourage readers to investigate these ideas as much as possible.

The Eight Diagrams represent the entire phenomenal world and in a unique way stimulate us to think less in a rational and factual manner and more in an intuitive imagery fashion. The Eight Diagrams and their associated symbolisms can be taken literally, as metaphors, or as archetypes. It is for this reason that they are so difficult to actually define. For example, should we think of Thunder *(Chen)* more as the natural reaction to lightning (an electrical discharge and vibration in the atmosphere)? Or should we look at it as to its effect or symbolic implications—"suddenness," "shaking," "excitement," "flashing," "stimulating," "arousing," "enlightenment," "quickening," and so on? In this work, however, the Eight Diagrams will, as much as possible, be dealt with purely in correlation to T'ai Chi Ch'uan.

There are few subjects in our world to which the Eight Diagrams could not be applied, whether it be family matters, affairs of governing, military strategy, business, alchemy, sexual congress, meditation, and so on. As the reader may perceive, it would be very difficult to elucidate the entire scope of these Eight Diagrams in any work, especially when discerning the additional interpretations and influences of King Wen's After Heaven arrangement, and the structuring of the sixty-four images.

As Confucius said about his study of the I Ching, "I regret not having another fifty years to study it."

THE EIGHT DIAGRAMS CORRELATION CHART

Many correlations have not been included here for lack of space. The following is an attempt to list the major correlations to show how extensive Chinese thought is concerning the Eight Diagrams.

SYMBOL & IMAGE	CONDITION	NATURE	PURPOSE	FUNCTION	FAMILY
Heaven	Creative	Strength	Ruling	Originating	Father
Earth	Receptive	Yielding	Storing	Devoting	Mother
Water	Abysmal	Perilous	Moistening	Injuring	Second Son
Fire	Clinging	Dependable	Drying	Exhibiting	Second Daughter
Wind	Gentleness	Penetrating	Scattering	Equaling	First Daughter
Thunder	Arousing	Inciting	Moving	Producing	First Son
Valley	Joyousness	Pleasuring	Coursing	Rejoicing	Youngest Daughter
Mountain	Keeping Still	Resting	Arresting	Completing	Youngest Son

SYMBOL & IMAGE	BODY	COLOR	SHAPE	OBJECTS	POSITIONS
Heaven	Head	Vermilion	Circles	Jade, Metal	Leader, Emperor
Earth	Stomach	Black	Squares	Cloth, Cauldron	Laborer, Minister
Water	Ears	Blood Red	Tubulars	Bow, Wheel	Robber, Subject
Fire	Eyes	Red Yellow	Spirals	Sword, Helmet	Soldier, Politician
Wind	Thighs	White	Horizontals	Carpenter's Square, Wood	Shopkeeper, Craftsman
Thunder	Feet	Azure Yellow	Verticals	Bamboo, Rushes	Entertainer, Philosopher
Valley	Mouth	Blue Green	Concaves	Sickle, Fields	Farmer, Concubine
Mountain	Hands	Azure	Convexes	Stones, Gateways	Servant, Eunuch

SYMBOL & IMAGE	EARTH ANIMAL	SPIRIT ANIMAL	MOON PHASE	DIRECTION	SEASON
Heaven	Horse	Dragon-Horse	New Moon	South	Summer
Earth	Ox	Unicorn	Full Moon	North	Winter
Water	Pig	White Snake	Half Moon (last ¼)	East	Spring
Fire	Pheasant	Magic Tortoise	Half Moon (first ¼)	West	Autumn
Wind	Birds, Fowl	Phoenix	Crescent (waning)	Northeast	Early Spring
Thunder	Yellow Dragon	Purple Dragon	Gibbous (waxing)	Southwest	Late Autumn
Valley	Sheep	Monkey King	Crescent (waxing)	Southeast	Later Summer
Mountain	Dog	Mountain Tiger	Gibbous (waning)	Northwest	Early Winter

SYMBOL & IMAGE	T'AI CHI POSTURE	EIGHT DEFECTS	EIGHT SKILLS	CH'I CAVITY	MERIDIAN
Heaven	Warding-Off	Opposing	Evading	Pai Hui	Tu Mo
Earth	Rolling-Back	Leaning	Returning	Hui Yin	Jen Mo
Water	Pressing	Discarding	Attaching	Shuang Kuan	Chuang Mo
Fire	Pushing	Resisting	Clearing	Chiang Kung	Tai Mo
Wind	Pulling	Severing	Circling	Yu Chen	Yin Wei Mo
Thunder	Splitting	Splicing	Changing	Ch'i Hai	Yin Chia Mo
Valley	Elbowing	Bending downward	Advancing	Kuan Hsuan	Yang Wei Mo
Mountain	Shouldering	Looking upward	Withdrawing	Ching Men	Yang Chia Mo

9 The After Heaven Arrangement of King Wen

The After Heaven arrangement of the Eight Diagrams, attributed to King Wen (Wen Wang) of the Chou dynasty, is not necessarily a different arrangement as such, but is to be viewed and used in conjunction with the Before Heaven arrangement. It is a means by which to see more clearly the workings of the Before Heaven arrangement, showing symbolically how each of the

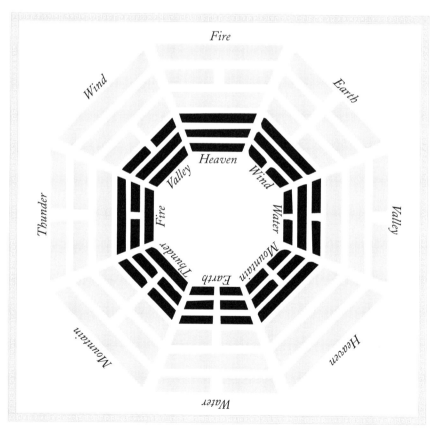

After Heaven arrangement (outer trigrams)
Before Heaven arrangement (inner trigrams)

Before Heaven images are reflected within our world. For example, the top-most image of the Before Heaven arrangement is Heaven, but King Wen places Fire in this position. The Fire image is located in this position because the aspects of actual fire (brightness, illumination, and so forth) reveal Heaven to us here on Earth, as Heaven is bright and illumining. King Wen arranged each of the Eight Diagrams in this manner, so that they reveal the inner quality and function of each image presented by Fu Hsi.

Below are some brief examples of how King Wen arranged the After Heaven images to work in conjunction with and to reflect Fu Hsi's Before Heaven arrangement.

Fire is the After Heaven condition of **Heaven,** as Heaven acquires light during its growth. Heaven is revealed by Fire because Fire represents brightness, which is the actual image coming forth from Heaven (the sun and sky). Without brightness and illumination there can be no Heaven. As for human beings, Fire and Heaven are the *Shen Ming*—the illumined or bright spirit.

Wind is the After Heaven condition of **Valley,** as wind carries the seeds of all the organisms and moves water for collection. Wind, therefore, reveals and maintains Valley. Water cannot flow and rain cannot fall without wind, as clouds must move with the wind to bring rain. A valley is an empty space through which the wind moves, just as our stomach is an empty vessel through which our breath moves.

Thunder is the After Heaven condition of **Fire,** as thunder brings light (lightning) and movement to brightness. Fire vibrates, hence Thunder reveals and creates Fire. Thunder is nature's source of natural fire. Without the idea of vibration, light cannot exist, such as when two sticks are rubbed together or two stones are struck against each other to create fire. Even the human body must create movement, internally and externally, in order to produce warmth—which is the idea behind "stimulating the *ch'i.*"

Mountain is the After Heaven condition of **Thunder,** as it is the shaking of Earth that produces mountains. The idea of the earth shaking, plates beneath the surface pushing upward and creating a mountain is what Thunder represents here. Without thunder the landscape could not exist. This is like the regenerative force rising into the head to activate the spirit.

Water is the After Heaven condition of **Earth,** as the earth acquires water during its growth. The earth is made up primarily of water, which is why our planet when seen from outer space appears blue. Water then reveals Earth, and without water there can be no Earth. The body of a human being is likewise comprised mostly of water.

Heaven is the After Heaven condition of **Mountain,** as mountains grow toward and reveal Heaven. Mountains are Heaven on Earth, and mountain tops have long been considered spiritual places, as heavenly abodes. Without mountains Earth would have no connection to Heaven. The head of our body is like a mountain, as it points to Heaven.

Valley is the After Heaven condition of **Water,** as water moves through valleys and low places. Valley therefore reveals Water because valleys collect bodies of water, such as oceans, seas, lakes, rivers, and streams. These channels, hollows, and valleys act as the conduits for the movement and collection of water, and are what make up the watery systems of the earth. The same is true for the organs and bloodstream within our body.

Earth is the After Heaven condition of **Wind,** as the earth creates conditions for wind to sustain itself. Wind is like the breath and custodian of Earth. Seeds of plants could not spread without wind, the waves of water systems would not move without wind, topsoil would not be dispersed without wind. Without wind the Earth would die of itself, just as our own body needs air to breathe.

10 The Philosophy of Before and After Heaven

In order to understand the basics of the two seemingly distinct arrangements of Fu Hsi and King Wen, you must first understand the Chinese concepts of Before Heaven and After Heaven. Once you understand these concepts, it is far easier to study and find meaning in the images and in their arrangements.

Prevalent in all Chinese thinking are the ideas of Before Heaven *(Hsien T'ien)* and After Heaven *(Hou T'ien)*. Even though these terms are used to define certain arrangements of the Eight Diagrams—the Fu Hsi (Before Heaven) and King Wen (After Heaven) arrangements—do not erroneously assume that they are the sole standard manner for defining the Eight Images. They not only apply themselves to the Eight Diagrams but they relate to many other ideas and expressions of thought as well.

Before Heaven, for example, can refer to the idea of what condition your spirit was in before you were born. After Heaven is then you as a living, material human being. Before Heaven can also mean the first half of your life and After Heaven the last half. It can also be said that Before Heaven is what existed before the creation of the Earth and After Heaven is the functioning of the Earth. Even our breath is considered by the Chinese in these terms. Before Heaven is the inhalation and After Heaven is the exhalation. The dialectics can be applied to everything, not just certain arrangements of the Eight Diagrams.

Primarily, Before Heaven means the condition of things at their origin, like when a baby is first conceived. This is the child's Before Heaven condition and is the product of his parents' genes and nature—their inherited qualities. The After Heaven condition is then the child growing into adulthood and being influenced by the outside world. The child's development stems mostly from experience and learning outside of the parents. Everything—whether it be the universe, our planet, each living being—must go through the process of Before and After Heaven conditions. So also must T'ai Chi, which is why the Before Heaven 16-Posture Form is based on the correlations of the Eight Images and the After Heaven 64-Posture Form is based on the sixty-four images of the I Ching.

We could go further and further with these correlations, but it will not be necessary for our purposes here. The question we can now answer is how the diagrams of the Before and After Heaven arrangements correlate to the Eight T'ai Chi Postures.

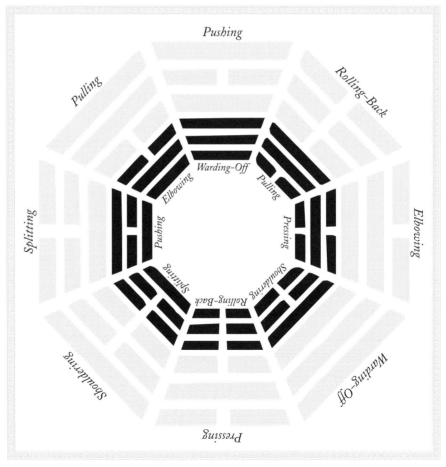

Eight Postures After Heaven arrangement (outer trigrams)
Eight Postures Before Heaven arrangement (inner trigrams)

To substantiate these correlations further, apart from their relationship to the Eight Diagram images and the T'ai Chi Posture Theory, I present the following translation of the *The Treatise on the Secrets of the Eight Postures*, one of the minor T'ai Chi Ch'uan treatises. All bracketed additions are mine.

TREATISE ON THE SECRETS OF THE EIGHT POSTURES

Warding-Off [Within Warding-Off there is Pushing]
What is the meaning of Warding-Off energy? It is like a boat floating on the water. Sink the *ch'i* into the *tan-t'ien,* then suspend the top of your head as if held by a string from above. The entire body should feel as if it had the releasing energy of a compressed spring [just like Pushing], instantly opening and closing. Even if confronted by a thousand pounds of incoming force, you could uproot and cause the opponent's root to float without any difficulty.

Rolling-Back [Within Rolling-Back there is Pressing]
What is the meaning of Rolling-Back energy? Entice the opponent to Advance [just like Pressing], follow his incoming energy, do not discard or resist it. When his strength is completely exhausted, he will naturally be empty. At this point you can let go or counter him [with Pressing]. Maintain your own Fixed-Rooting and no one can take advantage of you.

Pressing [Within Pressing there is Elbowing]
What is the meaning of Pressing energy? It functions in two ways: (1) The simplest is the direct method. Advance to meet [receive] the opponent, and then adhere and close in one action [just like Elbowing]. (2) To apply reaction force is the indirect method. This is like a ball bouncing off a wall or a coin tossed onto a drumhead, rebounding off with a ringing sound.

Pushing [Within Pushing there is Splitting]

What is the meaning of Pushing energy? When mobilizing this energy it is like flowing water. The substantial is concealed within the insubstantial [just like Splitting]. The force of a torrent is difficult to oppose. Reaching a high place, it swells and fills the entire space [just like Splitting]; coming into a low place it descends into it. There are troughs and crests within waves; there is no opening into which they cannot enter.

 Pulling [Within Pulling there is Rolling-Back]

What is the meaning of Pulling energy? It is like weighting a steel-yard beam. No matter how substantial or insubstantial the force is, the heaviness and lightness of it can be clearly distinguished [just like Rolling-Back]. To push or pull it requires but four ounces, yet a thousand pounds can be balanced on it. In asking what is the principle of this, the answer lies in the the function of the lever [just like Rolling-Back].

 Splitting [Within Splitting there is Shouldering]

What is the meaning of Splitting energy? Like a spinning disk when something is cast onto it, Splitting will immediately throw the opponent out more than ten feet [just like Shouldering]. Have you not seen a whirlpool, with its rolling torrent and spiraling currents? If leaves should fall in they are quickly dragged down it and disappear.

 Elbowing [Within Elbowing there is Pulling]

What is the meaning of Elbowing energy? The function is in the Five Activities.* The *yin* and *yang* are distinguished according to upper and lower [just like Pulling]. The substantial and insubstantial are to be clearly discriminated. If its motion is connected and unbroken, nothing can oppose its strength. The chopping of the fist is extremely fierce. After thoroughly understanding the Six Energies,** the functional use is unlimited.

---

*The Five Activities: Advancing, Withdrawing, Looking-Left, Gazing-Right, and Fixed-Rooting

**The Six Energies: Adhering, Sticking, Neutralizing, Seizing, Enticing, and Issuing

Shouldering [Within Shouldering there is Warding-Off]
What is the meaning of Shouldering energy? The method is
divided into the shoulder and back techniques. In Diagonal
Flying Posture [and Warding-Off] the shoulder is used, but
within the Shouldering Posture there is some use of the back.
Once you have the opportunity and positioning, the tech-
nique is like pounding a pestle. Pay attention to your Fixed-
Rooting. If you lose it, applying the technique will be in vain.

Other T'ai Chi treatises expound the ideas of the Illimitable *(Wu Chi)*,
the T'ai Chi symbol *(T'ai Chi T'u)*, the Two Powers of *yin* and *yang*
(Liang Szu), the Eight Diagrams *(Pa Kua)*, the Five Activities *(Wu*
Hsing), and the Three Powers *(San Tsai)*, but for our purposes here
they actually add no new revelations to what has already been dis-
cussed or will be presented later. The *Eight Gates and Five Steps*
Discourse, however, deserves a considerable amount of attention, as the
Eight Gates arrangement is a crucial element to forming the 16-
Posture and 64-Posture I Ching T'ai Chi Forms.

11 The Eight Gates Diagram

The Eight Gates and Five Steps Discourse is a T'ai Chi Ch'uan classical text that lists and associates the Eight Diagrams in a unique and different fashion from that of the Before Heaven and After Heaven arrangements, even though the Eight Gates works in conjunction with those arrangements. The relationship of the Five Steps (Five Activities), however, is the same as elsewhere presented, and needs no further discussion here.

Below is a comparative list showing how the Eight Diagrams correlate to the Eight Postures in the *T'ai Chi Ch'uan Treatise* and in the treatise on the Eight Gates and Five Steps. Before continuing on, I want to point out an error I corrected in the treatise. Whether this error was intentional (to hide its meaning) or simply an oversight is uncertain. The basis for the Eight Gates *(Pa Men)* in this discourse draws its correlations and structure from an older Eight Diagram arrangement derived from the Confucian classic *Li Chi (Book of Rites)*. In the *Book of Rites* the cosmology for the Eight Pillars of Heaven (Eight Diagrams) are correlated with the Eight Directions, or Eight Gates, which are the entrances from which the Eight Winds and rain clouds enter the atmosphere. *The Eight Gates and Five Steps Discourse,* however, contained a corruption by showing Thunder placed in the northern position and Fire in the western. To comply with the original arrangement expounded in the *Book of*

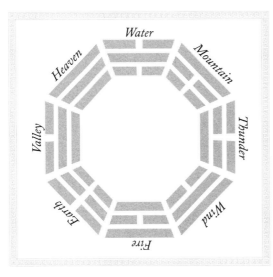

Eight Gates diagram

THE EIGHT GATES DIAGRAM

BH	POSTURE	DIRECTION	EIGHT GATES POSITIONING
1. Heaven, *Chien*	Warding-Off	South	Water, *K'an*, Pressing, South
2. Valley, *T'ui*	Elbowing	Southeast	Heaven, *Chien*, Warding-Off, Southeast
3. Fire, *Li*	Pushing	East	Valley, *T'ui*, Elbowing, East
4. Thunder, *Chen*	Splitting	Northeast	Earth, *K'un*, Rolling-Back, Northeast
5. Earth, *K'un*	Rolling-Back	North	Fire, *Li*, Pushing, North
6. Mountain, *Ken*	Shouldering	Northwest	Wind, *Sun*, Pulling, Northwest
7. Water, *K'an*	Pressing	West	Thunder, *Chen*, Splitting, West
8. Wind, *Sun*	Pulling	Southwest	Mountain, *Ken*, Shouldering, Southwest

Rites, however, their positions are reversed and presented in their correct positions here.

(EG = Eight Gates image, BH = Before Heaven image, AH = After Heaven image, CI = Complementary image. Bracketed additions are mine.)

In the *Book of Rites* the Eight Winds, or Pillars of Heaven, are described as follows:

1. From the South enter the storming winds and rain clouds [Water (EG), because of its position near Heaven (BH) and Fire (AH)].

2. From the Southeast enter the gentle winds and rain clouds [Heaven (EG), because of its position near Valley (BH) and Wind (AH)].

3. From the East enter the roaring winds and rain clouds [Valley (EG), because of its position near Fire (BH) and Thunder (AH)].

4. From the Northeast enter the burning winds and rain clouds [Earth (EG), because of its position near Thunder (BH) and Mountain (AH)].

5. From the North enter the cold winds and rain clouds [Fire (EG), because of its position near Earth (BH) and Water (AH)].

6. From the Northwest enter the sharp winds and rain clouds [Wind (EG), because of its position near Mountain (BH) and Heaven (AH)].

7. From the West enter the long lasting winds and rain clouds [Thunder (EG), because of its position near Water (BH) and Valley (AH)].

8. From the Southwest enter the cool winds and rain clouds [Mountain (EG), because of its position near Wind (BH) and Earth (AH)].

This Eight Gates arrangement is based on the natural interchanges and influences of Water, Heaven, Valley, Earth, Fire, Wind, Thunder, and Mountain upon their associated directions and BH and AH images. These stimulate and affect the movements of the Eight Winds and rain clouds, which can either be nourishing or damaging. The directions from which these all enter are called "gates." So in this arrangement, if Water enters (comes from) the southern gate (direction) with storming winds it can be damaging to Heaven (the sky filled with torrent winds and rains) or nourishing to Earth (the Earth needs rain to nourish itself). Each of the other Eight Winds can be viewed similarly.

Another aspect of the Eight Gates arrangement—which sounds complicated at first—the diagrams of the Eight Gates are derived from and act as the After Heaven diagrams of the Complementary Images, just as the After Heaveen diagrams are derived from the Before Heaven diagrams. For example, Water EG, which occupies Heaven's position in the Before Heaven arrangement, is the AH image of Earth BH, which is the Complementary image to Heaven BH. Examining the entire Eight Gate arrangement, the positioning of the images all follow this pattern—as the After Heaven images of the Before Heaven's Complementary images.

RELATING THE EIGHT GATES TO T'AI CHI

The arrangement of the Eight Gates in relation to T'ai Chi primarily shows that certain posture techniques can either establish or conquer other posture techniques. To view the conquering aspect, the EG image is shown in connection with its like-positioned BH image. To view the establishing aspect, the EG image is paired with the Complementary image of the like-positioned BH image. Examples of the conquering and establishing aspects for all of the Eight Gate images are presented.

1. Pressing (EG-Water) can conquer Warding-Off (BH-Heaven). Rolling-Back (CI-Earth) can establish Pressing.

2. Warding-Off (EG-Heaven) can conquer Elbowing (BH-Valley). Shouldering (CI-Mountain) can establish Warding-Off.

3. Elbowing (EG-Valley) can conquer Pushing (BH-Fire). Pressing (CI-Water) can establish Elbowing.

4. Rolling-Back (EG-Earth) can conquer Splitting (BH-Thunder). Pulling (CI-Wind) can establish Rolling-Back.

5. Pushing (EG-Fire) can conquer Rolling-Back (BH-Earth). Warding-Off (CI-Heaven) can establish Pushing.

6. Pulling (EG-Wind) can conquer Shouldering (BH-Mountain). Elbowing (CI-Valley) can establish Pulling.

7. Splitting (EG-Thunder) can conquer Pressing (BH-Water). Pushing (CI-Fire) can establish Splitting.

8. Shouldering (EG-Mountain) can conquer Pulling (BH-Wind). Splitting (CI-Thunder) can establish Shouldering.

THE FOUR LINEAR ARRANGEMENTS OF
THE EIGHT DIAGRAMS

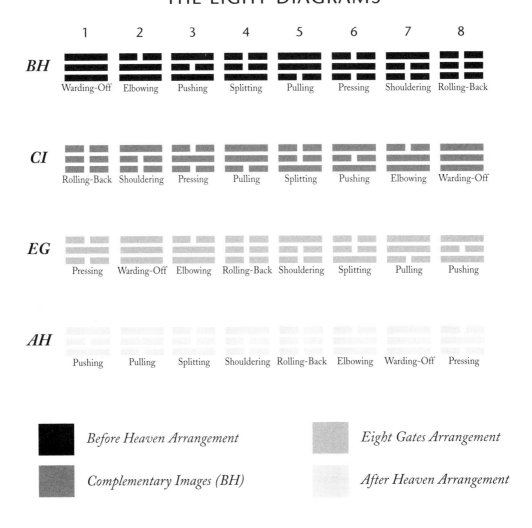

	1	2	3	4	5	6	7	8
BH	Warding-Off	Elbowing	Pushing	Splitting	Pulling	Pressing	Shouldering	Rolling-Back
CI	Rolling-Back	Shouldering	Pressing	Pulling	Splitting	Pushing	Elbowing	Warding-Off
EG	Pressing	Warding-Off	Elbowing	Rolling-Back	Shouldering	Splitting	Pulling	Pushing
AH	Pushing	Pulling	Splitting	Shouldering	Rolling-Back	Elbowing	Warding-Off	Pressing

Before Heaven Arrangement

Eight Gates Arrangement

Complementary Images (BH)

After Heaven Arrangement

By extension the entire process shown beforehand with just the images as indicated in the *Book of Rites* can be applied here to T'ai Chi postures. A great deal more could be discussed here, but it would take us much further and deeper into I Ching theory than is necessary. Those interested in working with this will discover that an incredible bulk of T'ai Chi theory can be created through the manipulation of images within this Eight Gates arrangement. But it is a most amazing configuration of natural development in I Ching theory, and without question is as ingenious and useful as King Wen's arrangement of the After Heaven images. The Eight Gates configuration and manner of interpreting the images are instrumental for viewing the natural progression of T'ai Chi postures. Therefore it was necessary to demonstrate to the reader the meaning and workings of the Eight Gates.

CIRCULAR DIAGRAM OF THE FOUR ARRANGEMENTS

Eight Diagram Theory

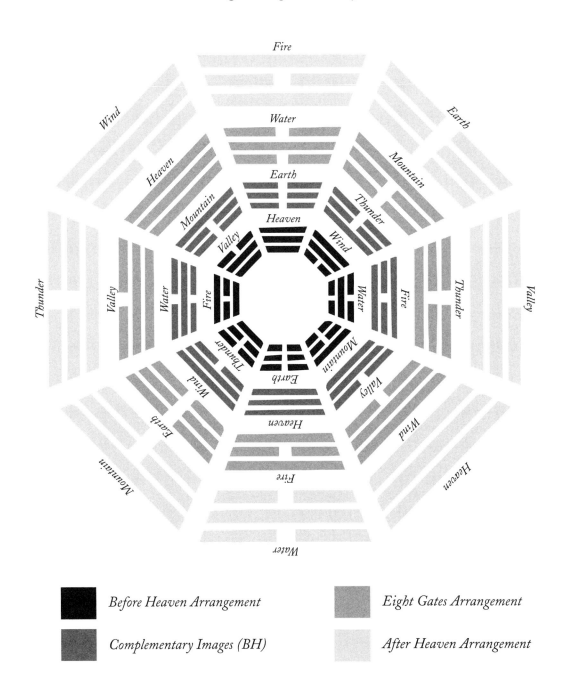

■ *Before Heaven Arrangement*

■ *Complementary Images (BH)*

■ *Eight Gates Arrangement*

□ *After Heaven Arrangement*

CIRCULAR DIAGRAM OF THE FOUR ARRANGEMENTS

T'ai Chi Posture Theory

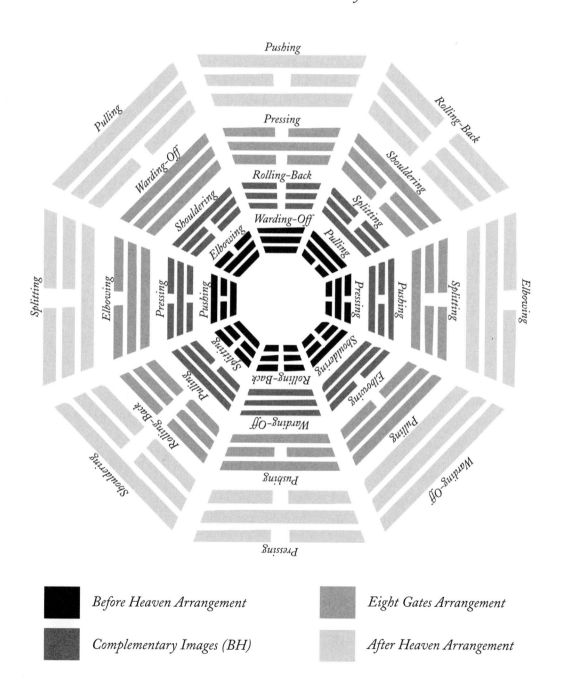

■ *Before Heaven Arrangement*		■ *Eight Gates Arrangement*
■ *Complementary Images (BH)*		■ *After Heaven Arrangement*

12 Developments of Wu Chi

Reproduced from Tung Ying-chieh's *Principles and Meanings of T'ai Chi Ch'uan*, the following graphic best shows the development of *Wu Chi* to T'ai Chi, the Two Powers *(Liang Szu)* of *yin* and *yang*, the Three Powers *(San Tsai)*, the Four Emblems *(Szu Hsiang)*, the Five Activities *(Wu Hsing)*, and the Eight Diagrams (Pa Kua). This development represents how all phenomena originally came into existence from nothingness, showing symbolically the theories presented in Lao Tzu's *Tao Te Ching* and later adopted into Taoism and T'ai Chi as well.

Although it is simple and concise, Tung's representation is extremely valuable for seeing the underlying philosophical elements of T'ai Chi in their relationship to each other.

Following Tung's graphic, I have added a circular chart showing how the major Chinese philosophical symbols developed from each other. The center image is *Wu Chi* and Earth (considered the center of all things in Chinese cosmology).

Even though they are not discussed in this book, I included the Twelve Animals because they are so prevalent in Chinese philosophy and geomancy, and so that readers who have an interest in Chinese astrology can see the relationship of the Twelve Animals to other I Ching symbols.

Wu Chi

極無

The entire being
is completely void.   全體透空   無形無象   Without any form,
without any image.

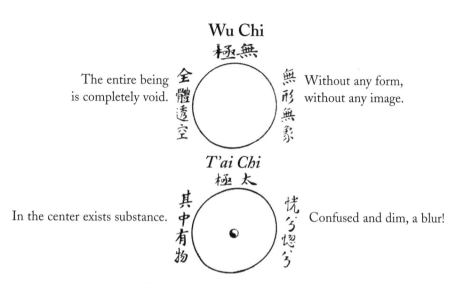

T'ai Chi

極太

In the center exists substance.   其中有物   恍兮惚兮   Confused and dim, a blur!

Two Powers and Three Powers

Motion and
tranquillity
wax and wane.
It is now complete
T'ai Chi *(San Tsai).*   乃成太極   動靜消長   判分陰陽   有餘不足   There is something,
but not yet sufficient.
Divides and separates
into *yin* and *yang*
(Liang I).

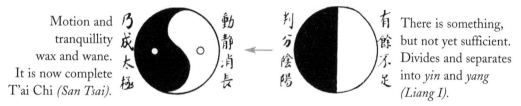

Four Emblems and Five Activities

行五象四

Winter and
Summer,
Spring and
Autumn,
bring about the
sojourning of the
Five Activities
(Wu Hsing).   寒暑以五行貞   10,000
Things
(Wan Wu)
return to Eartc
萬物歸於土   消長成老四象數   Waxing
and Waning,
old and young,
completely
evolving
into the
Four Emblems
(Szu Hsiang).

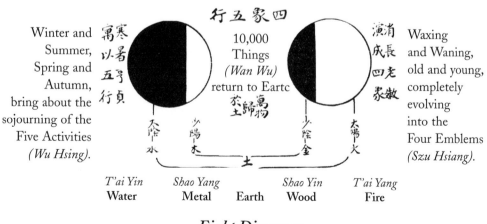

T'ai Yin	*Shao Yang*		*Shao Yin*	*T'ai Yang*
Water	**Metal**	**Earth**	**Wood**	**Fire**

Eight Diagrams

T'ai Yin *(Earth)*	*Shao Yin* *(Mountain)*	*Chung Yin* *(Water)*	*Lao Yin* *(Wind)*	*Lao Yang* *(Thunder)*	*Chung Yang* *(Fire)*	*Shao Yang* *(Valley)*	*T'ai Yang* *(Heaven)*

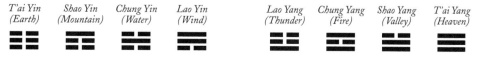

64 Images

CONCENTRIC SYMBOLIC REPRESENTATION OF THE TEN-THOUSAND THINGS

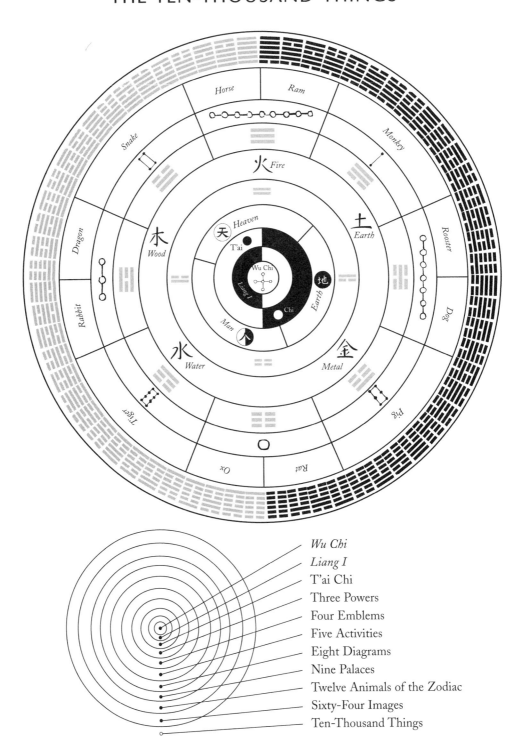

Wu Chi
Liang I
T'ai Chi
Three Powers
Four Emblems
Five Activities
Eight Diagrams
Nine Palaces
Twelve Animals of the Zodiac
Sixty-Four Images
Ten-Thousand Things

13 The Five Activities

(Wu Hsing)

Wu in Chinese means five; the term *Hsing* is much more difficult to define. The best, most concise definition explains it as "the constant state of change of elemental forces within being." Even though *Hsing* is normally translated as "agents," "attributes," "metamorphoses," or "elements," these are all aspects of *Hsing* and do not express the entire meaning. Because the idea of *Hsing* suggests forces in a constant state of change, I have chosen to use "activities" as the best singular term to express it.

In the chapter titled "Heng Fan" in the *Book of Documents* it says, "Water's function is to soak and descend; Fire's function is to burn and ascend; Wood's function is to curve and straighten; Metal's function is to obey and change; and Earth's function is to seed and harvest." From this brief statement, the list of correlations have swelled the bindings of many books.

The theory of the Five Activities saturates Chinese philosophy, probably even more so than the Eight Diagrams. One could hardly consider studying Chinese medical practices, geomancy, painting, music, craftsmanship, or even Taoism or Confucianism in any depth without a solid foundation in Five Activities theory. Hundreds of parallels can be made, and have been by the Chinese, concerning these five elemental forces of nature. My list of examples is very short considering how extensive it could be, but it should suffice for our purposes here. Many of the associations in the following chart come from the *Nei Ching*. The remainder come from a variety of other sources.

THE FIVE ACTIVITIES CHART

	Wood	Fire	Earth	Metal	Water
	Yang	*Yang*	Neutral	*Yin*	*Yin*
Direction	East	South	Center	West	North
Season	Spring	Summer		Autumn	Winter
Climate	Wind	Heat	Humidity	Dryness	Cold
Color	Green	Red	Yellow	White	Black
Organ	Liver	Heart	Spleen	Lungs	Kidneys
Orifice	Eyes	Ears	Nose	Mouth	Anus/genitals
Tissues	Ligaments	Arteries	Muscles	Skin/Hair	Bones
Flavor	Sour	Bitter	Sweet	Pungent	Salty
Odor	Rancid	Scorched	Fragrant	Rotten	Putrid
Emotion	Anger	Joy	Sympathy	Grief	Fear
Animal	Fowl	Sheep	Ox	Horse	Pig
Spiritual Animal	Dragon	Phoenix	Horse	Tiger	Tortoise
Grain	Wheat	Sticky Millet	Millet	Rice	Beans
Sound	Shouting	Laughing	Singing	Crying	Groaning
Spirit Force	*Hun* (Heaven)	*Shen* (Spirit)	*I* (Mind-Intent)	*P'o* (Earth)	*Chih* (Will)
Secretions	Perspiration	Mucous	Tears	Saliva	Sexual/urinary
Sexuality	Shy	Sensuous	Nourishing	Demanding	Passionate
Hour	3–7 A.M.	9 A.M.–1 P.M.	1–3, 7–9 A.M. & P.M.	3–7 P.M.	9 P.M.–1 A.M.
Heavenly Stems **—Yin Stem**	*I*	*Ting*	*Chi*	*Hsin*	*Kuei*
—Yang Stem	*Chia*	*Ping*	*Wu*	*Keng*	*Jen*
Earthly Branch	*Yin, Miao*	*Ssu, Wu*	*Ch'ou, Wei,* *Ch'en, Hsu*	*Shen, Yu*	*Tsu, Hai*
Diagram	Thunder, Wind	Fire	Mountain, Earth	Heaven, Valley	Water
T'ai Chi Posture	Splitting Pulling	Pushing	Shouldering, Rolling-Back	Warding-Off, Elbowing	Pressing
Activity	Withdrawing	Gazing-Right	Fixed-Rooting	Advancing	Looking-Left

One of the earliest and best treatments of the Five Activities was produced by Tung Chung-shu (179–104 B.C.E.), who belonged to the *Yin-Yang* School of Confucianism and wrote a brilliant treatise called *Ch'un Ch'iu Fan Lu (The Luxurious Gems of the Spring and Autumn Annals)*. Part of chapter forty-two, "The Meaning of the *Wu Hsing*," is provided below. The entire chapter is not pertinent, however, as much of it deals with Confucian associations on principles of benevolence and righteousness.

Tung Chung-shu was very Taoist in some of his thinking. He expounded that nature has great influence over man because the *yin* and *yang* forces are in both nature and man, and therefore man can have great influence over nature. This has a striking resemblance to what St. Augustine said—that there are no miracles, just unknown laws of nature. Tung was implying the same idea, for as powerful as nature can be over human beings, humans have power over nature through the knowledge and workings of *yin* and *yang*, which are in every sense the laws of nature.

Tung also believed that man is the miniature of the universe, the microcosm, and nature the macrocosm, which was very profound thinking for such a staunch Confucian. This idea was not new to Chinese thought, as it had previously been introduced by Buddhist thinkers, but it held many implications for Confucian thinkers because it lent itself so readily to Taoist views on man being but a small and insignificant factor of nature. Most Confucian ideology expounded that man was the mandate of Heaven, and Confucian society based itself on imitating Heaven, which they saw as a very organized and structured hierarchy. In every sense of the word, Heaven operated identically with human society, and it was the Son of Heaven (an emperor) who acted as the go-between for the two societies. Therefore, Tung, given his beliefs on the positions of nature and man (maybe unknowingly), expressed a very mystical and Taoist view on mankind and nature.

THE MEANING OF THE *WU HSING*
by Tung Chung-shu

Heaven has Five Activities: the first of which is Wood; the second Fire; the third Earth; the fourth Metal, and the fifth Water. Wood is the very source of the cycle of the Five Activities.

The natural cyclic sequence of these are that Wood produces Fire, Fire produces Earth, Earth produces Metal, Metal produces Water, and Water produces Wood—which is like the father and son relationship (each fathering their own offspring).

Wood sits to the left, Metal to the right, Fire in front, Water to the rear, and Earth occupies the middle.

These are like the order followed by father and son and the manner in which they (sons) receive (the genes of the father) and multiply (for posterity)—just as Wood receives from Water, Fire receives from Wood, Earth receives from Fire, Metal receives from Earth, and Water receives from Metal.

It is the Tao of Heaven that the son serve the father. Therefore, when Wood is produced, Fire must nourish it. When Metal perishes, Water should gather it. Fire enjoys Wood, nourishing it with *yang*. Water, however, overcomes Metal and buries it with *yin*. But only Earth serves Heaven with unconditional loyalty.

Wood controls production, Metal controls destruction, Fire controls heat, Water controls cold. Although Metal, Wood, Water, and Fire each have their own functions, their positions would not be possible were it not for Earth. Among the Five Activities and Four Seasons, Earth is included in all of them. The controlling factor of the Five Activities is the material force of Earth.

In T'ai Chi theory the application of the Five Activities is referred to in the *T'ai Chi Ch'uan Treatise* immediately following the correlation of the Eight Diagrams:

> Advancing, Withdrawing, Looking-Left, Gazing-Right, and
> Fixed-Rooting are then Metal, Wood, Water, Fire, and Earth.

The Five Activities, generally speaking, are the foundation of T'ai Chi movement and are associated with the feet in relation to the movements of the waist. The Eight Postures are associated with the hands in their relation to the waist. The T'ai Chi symbol represents the interchanging movements of *yin* and *yang* actions as they function at the waist. Therefore, the T'ai Chi symbol is commonly referred to as the T'ai Chi Waist, or the Function of T'ai Chi. The Five Activities are commonly referred to as the Foundation of T'ai Chi, and the Eight Postures as the Expression of T'ai Chi. From these associations, the Five Activities and Eight Postures, T'ai Chi was first named the Thirteen Postures. This use of the term "postures," however, was confusing and misleading, and so was dropped in favor of the name T'ai Chi Ch'uan. The confusion resulted from the fact that the Five Activities are aspects contained within the movements and expressions of each of the Eight Postures. They are the individual gesturings occurring within the execution of any of the Eight Postures.

In analogy, we can view the relationship between these three aspects according to the functioning of a wheel. The T'ai Chi symbol is like the axle upon which all the movements of the wheel rely. The Eight Postures are like the spokes that the entire wheel depends on for support. The Five Activities are like the rim of the wheel that provides the form on which the wheel can roll.

Another manner of viewing all this is to think of the T'ai Chi symbol as having two sides—one facing down, the other up. The Eight Diagrams, being the expression of the hands, develop upward from the symbol. The Five Activities being the foundation of the feet, develop downward. They both have associations with the center, the Function of the Waist (or T'ai Chi symbol), but since each has its own purpose they seem unrelated to each other. Just as the axle, spoke, and wheel may each appear as different forms and have different functions, together they work in harmony—and so it is with the T'ai Chi symbol, Eight Diagrams, and the Five Activities.

From the quote in the *T'ai Chi Ch'uan Treatise,* we see that Advancing is related to Metal, Withdrawing to Wood, Looking-Left to Water, Gazing-Right to Fire, and Fixed-Rooting to Earth. The theory of the Five Activities includes both the Creation and Destruction aspects of these five in relation to one another. In its Creation aspect, Metal produces Water, Water produces Wood, Wood produces Fire, Fire produces Earth, and Earth produces Metal. The Destruction is then, Metal destroys Wood, Wood destroys Earth, Earth destroys Water, Water destroys Fire, and Fire destroys Metal.

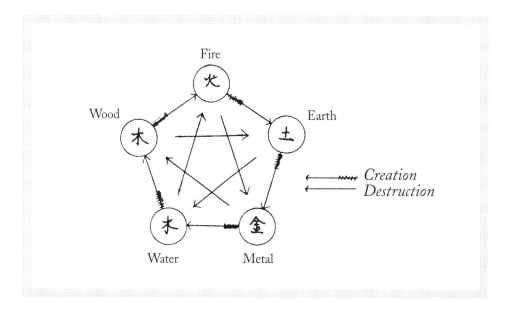

In relation to T'ai Chi activity, the above correlates the ideas that Advancing supports Looking-Left, Looking-Left supports Withdrawing, Withdrawing supports Gazing-Right, Gazing-Right supports Fixed-Rooting, and Fixed-Rooting supports Advancing. Conversely, Advancing hinders Withdrawing, Withdrawing hinders Fixed-Rooting, Fixed-Rooting hinders Looking-Left, Looking-Left hinders Gazing-Right, and Gazing-Right hinders Advancing.

Since Earth is central and embodies the other four elements of Metal, Water, Wood, and Fire, Fixed-Rooting is also embodied in each of the actions of Advancing, Withdrawing, Looking-Left, and Gazing-Right.

The Five Activities developed and are correlated from the production and symbolism of T'ai Chi (the *Ta-I* or *T'ai I,* the Great Oneness, of *yin* and *yang*), which represented Earth (as it embodies the other Four Elements). Fire, Metal, Wood, and Water represent Greater *(T'ai) Yang,* Lesser *(Shao) Yang,* Lesser *(Shao) Yin,* and Greater *(T'ai) Yin,* respectively. Just as T'ai Chi embodies and produces the Four Emblems, *Szu Hsiang* (see illustration on page 85).

In the minor T'ai Chi Ch'uan classical texts we find the *Treatise on the Songs of the Five Methods:*

TREATISE ON THE VERSES OF THE FIVE METHODS

Verse of Advancing

When there is an opportunity for Advancing, do so without hesitation. When encountering no obstacles, keep Advancing. Failing to Advance at the proper moment, the opportunity will be lost. If you seize the opportunities for Advancing, you can always be victorious.

Verse of Withdrawing

Stepping must be in accordance with the movements of the entire body. Then the technique will be without defect. Avoid the Substantial and seek the Insubstantial, then the opponent's attack will land on emptiness. Failing to Withdraw when the need arises for retreat is neither wise nor brave. Withdrawing is Advancing, as it must be changed into a counteroffensive.

Verse of Looking-Left

Whether the attack is from the left or right, the *yin* and *yang* aspects must change according to each circumstance. When neutralizing to the left, strike from the right with firmly rooted steps. The hands and feet function in unison, as do the knees, elbows, and waist. If performed correctly, the opponent will be unable to apprehend your actions and will find no recourse for defense.

Verse of Gazing-Right

With a false intent to the left, the true attack comes from the right with resolute stepping. Whether attacking to the right or to the left, the opportunities must be taken advantage of. Avoid the front and move to the side, then a superior position can be gained. Left and right, Substantial and Insubstantial, there can be no error in this method.

Verse of Fixed-Rooting*

Be centered, rooted, and still as a mountain. Sink the *ch'i* into the *tan-t'ien,* and be as if suspended from above. Gather the spirit of vitality within and relax the outward appearance. When either Receiving or Issuing,** they each must be performed instantly.

---

* The term Fixed-Rooting is sometimes referred to as Central Equilibrium. The differences come from whether or not the Chinese character for *Ting* is compounded with *Chung* (Central). *Chung Ting* is also used to mean the Central Fixed Position of the T'ai Chi symbol, so it invariably gets confused with just Fixed-Rooting *(ting)* of the Five Activities.

** Receiving and Issuing refer to the intrinsic energies developed in T'ai Chi martial arts training exercises.

14 The Three Powers

(San Tsai)

In Chinese philosophy, the concept that all things are related to the Three Powers of Heaven, Earth, and Man predominates almost all philosophical traditions. Here are some example subjects classified under the Three Powers:

Heaven	*Earth*	*Man*
Tao	*Virtue*	*Humanity*
Father	*Mother*	*Child*
Shen	*Ch'i*	*Ching*
Mind	*Breath*	*Body*
Penis	*Vagina*	*Fluids*
Spiritual	*Worldly*	*Humanistic*
Ruler	*Minister*	*Subject*
Function	*Form*	*Substance*
Upper	*Middle*	*Lower*
T'ai	*Chi*	*Ch'uan*
Movement	*Stillness*	*Intent*
Teacher	*Method*	*Student*
Happiness	*Prosperity*	*Longevity*
Circle	*Square*	*Line*

SAN TSAI DIAGRAM

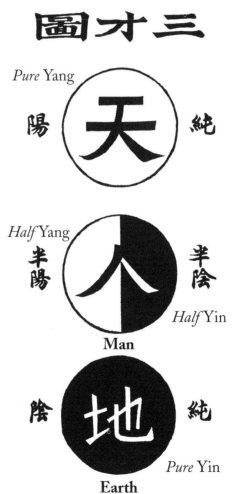

The following information describes how the concept of the Three Powers is interrelated to the T'ai Chi symbol, lines of the images, and the images themselves. Please refer to the *Treatise on the Eight Diagrams,* Eighth Wing, in which these associations were first developed and mentioned.

T'ai Chi Symbol (T'ai Chi T'u):

The white, left side represents Heaven. The right, dark side represents Earth. The small white and dark circles in each opposite side represent Man.

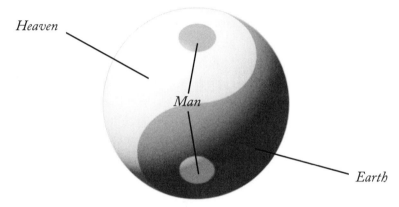

Lines (Yao):

In the Eight Diagrams each image has three lines. The top line is Heaven, the middle line is Earth, and the bottom line is Man. In the six-line images of the sixty-four images, the top two lines are Heaven, the middle two are Earth, and the bottom two are Man.

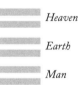

Images (Kua):

In the Eight Diagrams, the Heaven and Earth images represent themselves and the other six images represent Man.

Before Heaven images represent Heaven:
Shen (Spirit and the Mind).

Complementary images represent Earth:
Ch'i (Vital Energy and the Breath).

Eight Gates and After Heaven images represent Man:
Ching (Sexual Energy and the Body).

Three Powers (San Tsai)

The Way of Heaven is determined by distinguishing
the lines or images as *yin* and *yang*.

The Way of Earth is determined by distinguishing
the lines or images as Yielding and Unyielding.

The Way of Man is determined by distinguishing
the lines or images as Virtue and Humanity.

The term "Man" needs further clarification, as the heading of Man is never
viewed in a singular sense. In the Three Powers, the Man aspects must be seen
in their dualistic sense. Man can either be male or female. This is shown in the
T'ai Chi symbol in which the small white and dark circles represent Man, but
the white circle is specifically symbolic of males, and the dark circle symbolic
of females. Just as in Father, Mother, and Child, the Child can be either male
or female. The term Man is expressed singularly, but is meant to be dualistic.
Two other examples will help clarify this idea. In Penis, Vagina, and Fluids,
the Fluids can either be those of males or females, or of both—male secretions,
female secretions, or sperm and egg. In the example of Movement, Stillness,
and Intent, the Intent can be either "to move" or "to be still."

In connection with the 16-Posture I Ching T'ai Chi Form, each posture is
associated with its Before Heaven, Complementary, Eight Gates, and After
Heaven images—and each of these four images is further correlated with the
Three Powers. The Before Heaven images represent the Power of Heaven, the
Complementary images the Power of Earth, and the Eight Gates and After
Heaven images the Power of Man. In this way the application, progression,
and changes for each posture can be seen and determined clearly. Explanations
of the four images associated with each posture are provided in part 3—see
also the Four Arrangements charts on pages 82–83.

As an example, the Three Powers representations for Pressing, the fourth
T'ai Chi posture, are correlated to the following four images (see chart on
pages 100 and 101 for the other fifteen postures):

The Before Heaven image for Pressing is Water.
Water then represents the first power of *Heaven*.

The Complementary image for Water is Fire,
which lies opposite of Water in the Before Heaven arrangement.
Fire then represents the second power of *Earth*.

The Eight Gates image for Water is Thunder
(as Thunder is the After Heaven representation for Fire—
the Complementary image to Water).
The After Heaven image for Water is Valley.
Thunder and ***Valley*** then represent the third power of *Man*.

By knowing the four diagram images for Pressing, the Three Powers correlations to the corresponding T'ai Chi postures can also be made:

The Before Heaven image of *Pressing*
represents the first power of *Heaven*.

Pushing, Pressing's Complement,
represents the second power of *Earth*.

Splitting and Elbowing, Pushing and Pressing's
After Heaven images, **represent the third power of Man.**

In T'ai Chi terms, Pressing (Water) naturally leads to Pushing (Fire), as Pushing is the Complement of Pressing, and within Pressing there is the intent and possibility of change for Splitting (Thunder) and Elbowing (Valley)—just as Thunder (vibration) is visible in Fire, and Water is seen in the Valley. Each posture can be viewed and determined in such a manner. Conversely, Splitting and Elbowing could change to Pressing, and Pressing can change to Pushing.

In terms of inner cultivation, the preceding example shows the images of Water (which represents *ching*) and Fire (which represents *ch'i*) creating Thunder within the Valley (which represents the abdomen, or the cauldron—the Taoist representation of where the spirit *[shen]* unites with the *ching* and *ch'i* to refine the Elixir.

These types of correlations can be made throughout all the T'ai Chi postures and with their corresponding images as well.

The following chart shows the relationship of the Three Powers of Heaven, Earth, and Man for each of the sixteen postures of the Before Heaven I Ching T'ai Ch'i Form.

THREE POWERS CHART OF
THE 16-POSTURE I CHING T'AI CHI FORM

	HEAVEN		**EARTH**		**MAN**		
Posture Name	*Before Heaven*		*Complementary*		*Eight Gates*		*After Heaven*
1. *Beginning T'ai Chi Posture*	*Water* (K'an) *Pressing*		*Fire* (Li) *Pushing*		*Thunder* (Chen) *Splitting*		*Valley* (T'ui) *Elbowing*
2. *Warding-Off, Left and Right*	*Heaven* (Chien) *Warding-Off*		*Earth* (K'un) *Rolling-Back*		*Water* (K'an) *Pressing*		*Fire* (Li) *Pushing*
3. *Rolling-Back*	*Earth* (K'un) *Rolling-Back*		*Heaven* (Chien) *Warding-Off*		*Fire* (Li) *Pushing*		*Water* (K'an) *Pressing*
4. *Pressing*	*Water* (K'an) *Pressing*		*Fire* (Li) *Pushing*		*Thunder* (Chen) *Splitting*		*Valley* (T'ui) *Elbowing*
5. *Pushing*	*Fire* (Li) *Pushing*		*Water* (K'an) *Pressing*		*Valley* (T'ui) *Elbowing*		*Thunder* (Chen) *Splitting*
6. *Single Whip*	*Wind* (Sun) *Pulling*		*Thunder* (Chen) *Splitting*		*Mountain* (Ken) *Shouldering*		*Earth* (K'un) *Rolling-Back*
7. *Lifting Hands*	*Thunder* (Chen) *Splitting*		*Wind* (Sun) *Pulling*		*Earth* (K'un) *Rolling-Back*		*Mountain* (Ken) *Shouldering*
8. *Shouldering*	*Mountain* (Ken) *Shouldering*		*Valley* (T'ui) *Elbowing*		*Wind* (Sun) *Pulling*		*Heaven* (Chien) *Warding-Off*

HEAVEN   EARTH   MAN

Posture Name	Before Heaven	Complementary	Eight Gates	After Heaven
9. White Crane Spreads Wings	Valley (T'ui) Elbowing	Mountain (Ken) Shouldering	Heaven (Chien) Warding-Off	Wind (Sun) Pulling
10. Brush Knee and Twist Step	Wind (Sun) Pulling	Thunder (Chen) Splitting	Mountain (Ken) Shouldering	Earth (K'un) Rolling-Back
11. Playing the Guitar	Thunder (Chen) Splitting	Wind (Sun) Pulling	Earth (K'un) Rolling-Back	Mountain (Ken) Shouldering
12. Chop with Fist	Water (K'an) Pressing	Fire (Li) Pushing	Thunder (Chen) Splitting	Valley (T'ui) Elbowing
13. Deflect, Parry, and Punch	Fire (Li) Pushing	Water (K'an) Pressing	Valley (T'ui) Elbowing	Thunder (Chen) Splitting
14. Follow to Seal, Carry to Close	Heaven (Chien) Warding-Off	Earth (K'un) Rolling-Back	Water (K'an) Pressing	Fire (Li) Pushing
15. Crossing Hands	Earth (K'un) Rolling-Back	Heaven (Chien) Warding-Off	Fire (Li) Pushing	Water (K'an) Pressing
16. Conclusion of T'ai Chi	Fire (Li) Pushing	Water (K'an) Pressing	Valley (T'ui) Elbowing	Thunder (Chen) Splitting

PART III

The Before Heaven Form

With the Images and the Philosophy

15 The 16-Posture I Ching T'ai Chi Form Arrangement

Having developed and presented the framework of the *I Ching T'ai Chi* style, the 16-Posture I Ching T'ai Chi Form can now be exclusively discussed and shown. My hope is that the previous material has sufficiently explained many of the underlying aspects of T'ai Chi and its relationship to I Ching imagery and Taoist philosophy.

Two items must be factored in to determine the sequence of the Before Heaven 16-Posture Form:

1. The Eight Postures of Warding-Off, Rolling-Back, and so on are to be matched to their corresponding images as mentioned in the *T'ai Chi Ch'uan Treatise.*
2. The first posture, or movement, has to represent the image of Water and the last posture Fire, which is a condition set down in the I Ching itself with the images #63 and #64, After Completion and Before Completion. As in the 64-Posture I Ching T'ai Chi Form, the process of inner cultivation involves bringing Fire below Water, so to heat the fluids, or *ching,* and mobilize the *ch'i.* Therefore, the *16-Posture Form* concludes by bringing Fire under Water.

Posture #1, Beginning T'ai Chi, therefore, is predetermined to be Water and Posture #16, Conclusion of T'ai Chi, to be Fire—Water's Complement. Posture #2, Warding-Off, follows according to the correlations of the *T'ai Chi Ch'uan Treatise,* which lists the postures in the sequence of Heaven (Warding-Off), Earth (Rolling-Back), Water (Pressing), Fire (Pushing), Wind (Pulling), Thunder (Splitting), Valley (Elbowing), and Mountain (Shouldering)—however, for reasons to be explained shortly, Mountain (Shouldering) comes before Valley (Elbowing).

The second posture then is Warding-Off, the third Rolling-Back, the fourth Pressing, the fifth Pushing, and so on. The first eight postures, concluding with Shouldering, are the *yang* Before Heaven postures, the ninth through sixteenth postures are the *yin* After Heaven postures or we could likewise say the first half of the form is Before Heaven and the second half, After Heaven. The eighth posture, Shouldering (Mountain), naturally transitions into the ninth posture of White Crane Spreading Wings—Valley (Mountain's Complement), so that the form follows not only the *T'ai Chi Ch'uan Treatise*, but moves from Fixed Images to their Complements, from *yang* postures into *yin*, and from Before Heaven into After Heaven.

We can now address the change in the sequential order of the Valley and Mountain images. These are reversed in the 16-Posture Form—with Mountain (Shouldering) placed first and Valley (Elbowing) coming after it—to comply with the workings of the T'ai Chi symbol itself. Within *yang* there is *yin*, and within *yin* there is *yang*. In this case, Valley represents the *yang* within the *yin* movements, and Mountain represents the *yin* within the *yang* movements. The chart on the following page clearly shows their positionings.

Also, as explained in the *Treatise on the Eight Diagrams* (see page 66), "Mountains and Valleys were to interchange their influences on each other." Again, because Mountain and Valley represent the *yin* and *yang* of the T'ai Chi symbol, the I Ching here clearly calls for their interchange in the arrangement, the natural logic in calculating the sequence of the 16-Posture Form. Interestingly, every T'ai Chi style performs Shouldering (Mountain) before Elbowing (Valley) and never provides an explanation for doing so. But the proper sequence and order of Warding-Off, Rolling-Back, Pressing, Pushing, Pulling, and Splitting is always found—no matter what posture names are given in the various styles; their intents are identical with the Eight Postures. In only this one regard, Shouldering preceding Elbowing, is the common order disturbed.

The Before Heaven Form has sixteen postures because of applying Complementary images. Postures #1 and #16, then, are complementary images, as are #2 and #15, #3 and #14, #4 and #13, #5 and #12, #6 and #11, #7 and #10, and #8 and #9. The arrangement of the images works in on itself, just as the *yin* and *yang* aspects of the T'ai Chi symbol turn in on themselves to provide eight *yang* Before Heaven postures and eight *yin* After Heaven postures.

CHART OF THE *BEFORE HEAVEN* 16-POSTURE FORM WITH CORRESPONDING TRIGRAMS

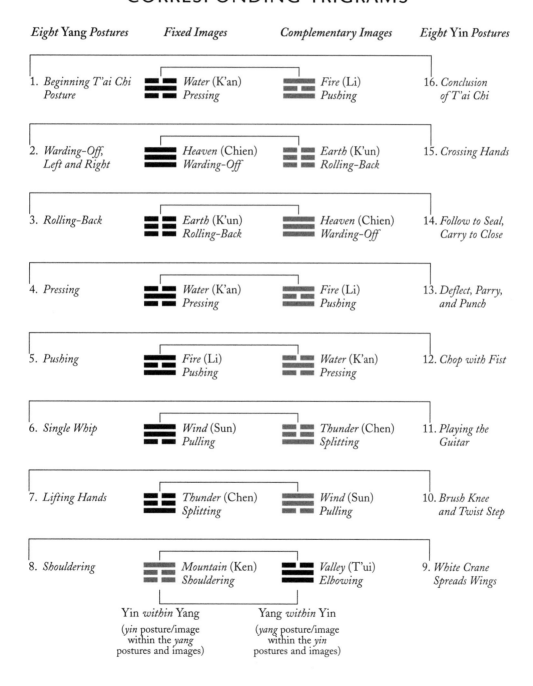

Eight Yang *Postures*   *Fixed Images*   *Complementary Images*   *Eight* Yin *Postures*

1. *Beginning T'ai Chi Posture* — *Water (K'an) Pressing* — *Fire (Li) Pushing* — 16. *Conclusion of T'ai Chi*

2. *Warding-Off, Left and Right* — *Heaven (Chien) Warding-Off* — *Earth (K'un) Rolling-Back* — 15. *Crossing Hands*

3. *Rolling-Back* — *Earth (K'un) Rolling-Back* — *Heaven (Chien) Warding-Off* — 14. *Follow to Seal, Carry to Close*

4. *Pressing* — *Water (K'an) Pressing* — *Fire (Li) Pushing* — 13. *Deflect, Parry, and Punch*

5. *Pushing* — *Fire (Li) Pushing* — *Water (K'an) Pressing* — 12. *Chop with Fist*

6. *Single Whip* — *Wind (Sun) Pulling* — *Thunder (Chen) Splitting* — 11. *Playing the Guitar*

7. *Lifting Hands* — *Thunder (Chen) Splitting* — *Wind (Sun) Pulling* — 10. *Brush Knee and Twist Step*

8. *Shouldering* — *Mountain (Ken) Shouldering* — *Valley (T'ui) Elbowing* — 9. *White Crane Spreads Wings*

Yin *within* Yang
(*yin* posture/image within the *yang* postures and images)

Yang *within* Yin
(*yang* posture/image within the *yin* postures and images)

The Ten T'ai Chi Stances

T'ai Chi movements contain ten basic stances, or footwork, which are the positionings of the feet and legs in conjunction with the waist. These stances are extremely important and must be practiced so that they can be performed without any error, as the feet and legs are the very foundation and function of T'ai Chi movement. If the footwork is sloppy and incorrect, so will be the T'ai Chi movements. The Ten T'ai Chi Stances all relate to the functions of the Five Activities and Five Operations.

THE FIVE ACTIVITIES

Advancing: to shift, sink, or step forward
Withdrawing: to shift, sink, or step backward
Looking-Left: to turn or shift leftward
Gazing-Right: to turn or shift rightward
Fixed-Rooting: after any movement the body must be relaxed
    and the rootedness in the feet must constantly be reestablished

THE FIVE OPERATIONS

Two types of *Rising:* rear leg and front leg—with the body
    facing any of the Eight Directions
Two types of *Sinking:* rear leg and front leg—with the body
    facing any of the Eight Directions
Four types of *Shifting:* forward, backward, leftward,
    or rightward
Two types of *Turning:* left and right
Five types of *Stepping:* stepping forward, stepping back,
    stepping left, stepping right, and Repositioning Step
    (Slide Step or Change Step*)

---

* Repositioning Steps occur in Sword, Sabre, and Staff practices and in Sensing Hands *(T'ui-Shou)*, Rolling-Back Hands *(Ta-Lu)*, and Dispersing Hands *(San-Shou)* training methods. They are not used within the Before and After Heaven forms.

1. *Riding a Horse Stance*

The original name of this posture was Sitting on a Horse Stance *(Tso Ma P'u)*. The name Riding a Horse is very descriptive, and should need no comment. It is also sometimes referred to as Bestriding the Horse Stance. The feet are positioned at shoulders' width, which is the Middle Position for horse stances. There is also the Extended Position, with the feet held one foot-length farther apart than shoulders' width, and the Narrow Position, where the feet are held at just one foot-length apart. In the *16-Posture I Ching T'ai Chi Form,* only the Middle Position is used.

In the Riding a Horse Stance it is also important to position both feet so that the toes are pointing straight ahead. Drawing in the *wei lu* (tailbone) cavity is also critical, so that the spine does not lean forward and the buttocks do not protrude.

There are three weight distribution placements of this stance—equal weight (which only occurs in the *Wu Chi,* Beginning, and Concluding postures—in which case the stance is referred to as Seated Horse) and the majority of the weight shifted into either the right or left leg. The body must be slightly sunk in these stances.

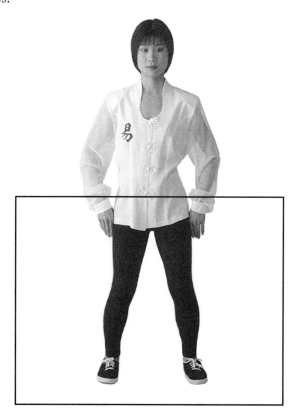

2. *Bow and Arrow Stance*

The original name of this stance was Supporting Stance *(Tien P'u)*. The name Bow and Arrow comes from the image of a man standing with a drawn bow ready to release an arrow. There are both right and left styles, which are indicated by the forward leg. The proper positioning of this stance is for the feet to be two foot-lengths or shoulders' width apart. The forward leg should be three foot-lengths to the front. The front foot, specifically the toes, is pointed directly ahead. The foot has a natural curve, so if the toes point straight ahead, the buttocks will be slightly pinched and will obstruct the *hui yin* cavity, located in the perineum area. The rear foot is turned out at a 45-degree angle. The majority of the weight (70 percent or so) is in the front leg, and the rear leg retains about 30 percent. The knee of the front leg is not to go beyond the toes, but this does not mean that the kneecap lines up with the toe tips, rather that the shin and calf are positioned perpendicularly, and if looking down, you are able to see the toes. The body in this stance is slightly sunk.

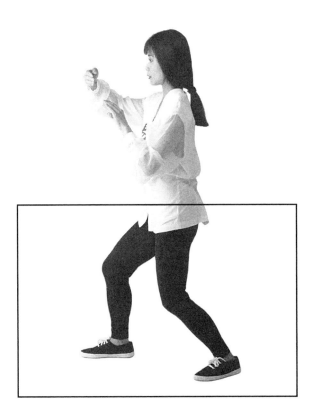

3. *Seated Tiger Stance*

This stance has had two earlier names, Empty or Insubstantial Stance *(Hsu P'u)*. It has also been called the Preying Tiger and the Crouching Tiger, and sometimes simply the Cat Stance. This stance, Seated Tiger, supposedly imitates a tiger ready to pounce on its prey, with one paw extended to the front and held slightly off the ground so that it can either seize with it or leap outward onto its prey. The positioning of this stance is for all the weight to be in the rear leg, with the foot turned out about 60 degrees. The front-leg toes are rested on the ground about two foot-lengths to the front and one foot-length over in width. Again, it is important to draw in the *wei lu* and keep the back straight when performing this stance. The rear leg must be slightly bent. There can be either a left or right style, indicated by the rear leg.

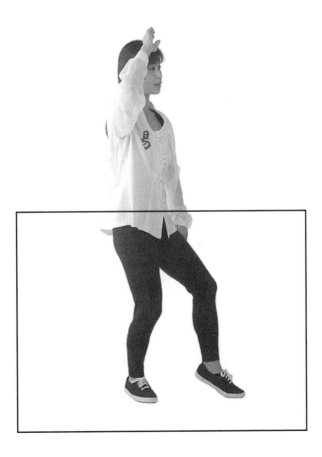

4. *Seven Star Stance*

The original name of this stance was Treading Stance *(T'a P'u)*. The name Seven Star comes from the image of the seven stars of the Big Dipper, Ursa Major, constellation. It was later applied to the seven days of the week. The weight is placed entirely in the rear leg and the front-foot heel is placed on the ground about two foot-lengths to the front and one foot-length over in width. Again, this stance requires special attention to drawing in the *wei lu* and straightening the back. The rear leg must be slightly bent. There can be either a left or right style, indicated by the rear leg.

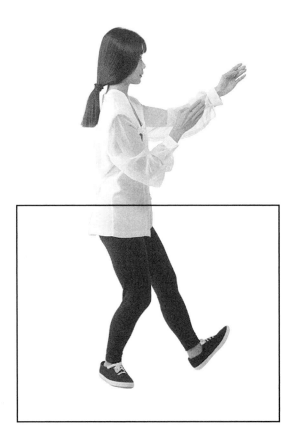

5. *Climbing a Mountain Stance*

This stance was originally called Rear Supporting Stance *(Hou Tien P'u)*. The name Climbing a Mountain derives from the image of someone climbing up a mountainside, where one must push off of the back leg in order to advance. The weight is placed entirely in the rear leg, and the front foot is placed flat on the ground with two foot-lengths to the front and shoulders' width apart. This stance requires special attention to the principle of suspending the head. There is both a left and right style, indicated by the rear leg.

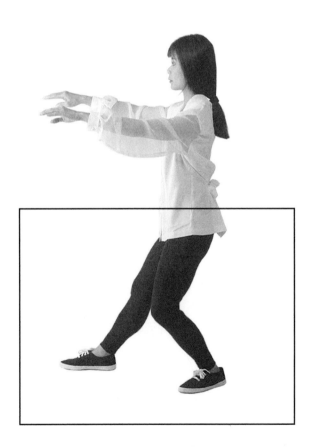

6. *Golden Rooster Stance*

Originally called Separating the Body Stance *(Fen Shen P'u)*. The Golden Rooster is symbolic of the sun and is also called the Golden Crow. The full name of this stance, like the After Heaven I T'ai Chi Form posture, is Golden Rooster Standing on One Leg. All the weight is placed on one leg, and the other is raised off the ground with the thigh held level and the foot held parallel to the ground. There are both left- and right-style stances, indicated by the standing leg. The principles of suspending the head and hollowing the chest are important in this stance.

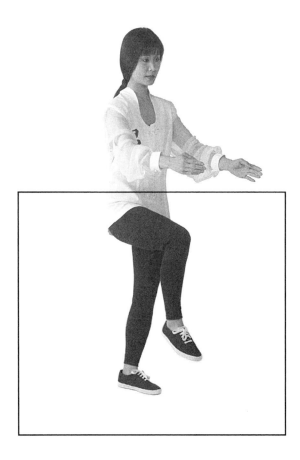

7. *Eight Shape Stance*

Originally called Joining the Branches Stance *(Lien Chih P'u)*. The name of this stance is a reference to the Chinese character for *pa,* meaning eight. The stance can be executed with the weight either in the front leg or rear leg. The rear leg is positioned at an outward 45-degree angle, the front leg is positioned two or three foot-lengths to the front and one foot-length width or even shoulders' width apart. There are both left and right styles, indicated by the front leg.

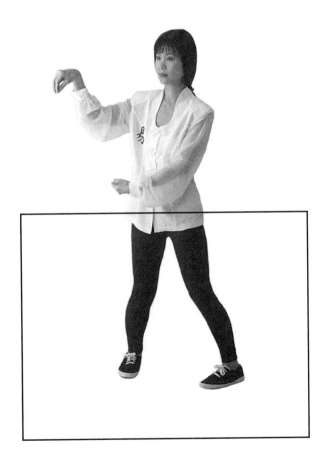

8. *Twisting Dragon Stance*

This posture is also called Binding Flowers Stance *(Chiao Hua P'u)*. The name Twisting Dragon is symbolic of a dragon twisting around a pillar. In the rightward style, the weight is placed in the front, right leg, with the foot turned out 45 degrees. The rear foot is held lightly to the ground and the waist is turned toward the right and the body is sunk low. The width is three foot-lengths to the front, and the rear leg is shoulders' width apart. The leftward style is opposite of this. Pay special attention to the principles of sinking the shoulders and drawing in the *wei lu*.

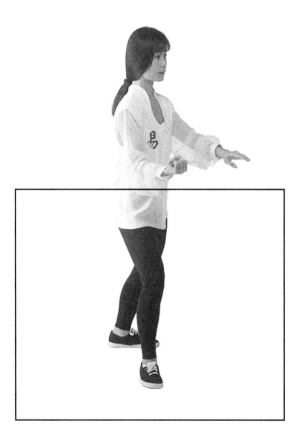

9. *Crawling Snake Stance*

This stance was originally called Grinding-Mill Stance *(Nien P'u)*. The image of a crawling snake is to indicate the low squatting position of the stance and the turning gestures within the movements of the After Heaven I T'ai Chi posture Snake Glides Downward. All the weight is placed in the rear leg, with the foot turned out 90 degrees. The front foot has very little weight placed on it and is also turned 90 degrees. There are left and right styles, indicated by the rear leg. In this stance attention must be paid to the principles of suspending the head and sinking the shoulders.

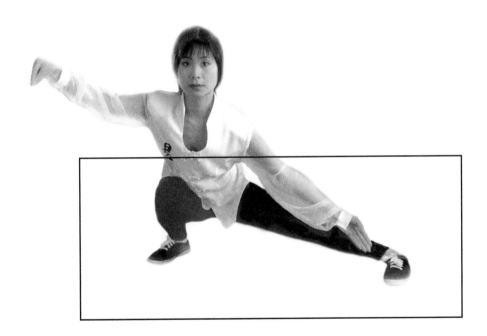

10. *Immortal Stance*

Originally called Fishing on a Horse Stance *(Tiao Ma P'u)*. The name of this stance, Immortal, is to represent the image of an immortal standing atop a precipice overlooking the valley below. The majority of the weight is placed in the front leg, and about 30 percent in the rear leg. The stance looks like a cross between the Riding a Horse and Bow and Arrow stances. The front leg is one foot-length in front of the rear leg, and the rear leg is at shoulders' width. There are left- and right-style stances indicated by the front leg. Pay special attention to the principles of drawing in the *wei lu* and raising the back.

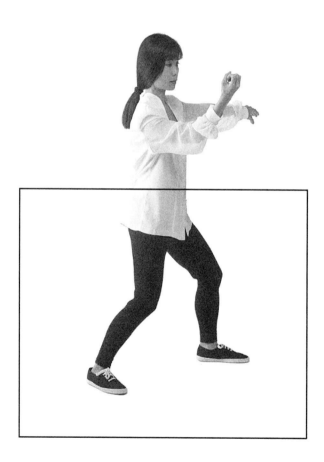

The Eight Hands

In T'ai Chi the Eight Diagrams symbolize the Eight Postures, and these Eight Postures are the techniques and positionings of the torso, arms, and hands. These Eight *Yin-Yang* Hands are then the expression of T'ai Chi movements and postures, also simply called Eight Hands *(Pa Shou)*. The Five Activities, in kind, represent the feet and legs. In the T'ai Chi system of practice, the empty-hand forms—Before and After Heaven forms, T'ai Chi Ch'i-Kung, Sensing Hands *(T'ui-Shou)*, Rolling-Back Hands *(Ta Lu)*, and Dispersing Hands *(San-Shou)*—all share the arrangement and indications of the following Eight *Yin-Yang* Hands. The T'ai Chi Sword practice has its own distinct patterns and positionings of the Eight Hands, as do the T'ai Chi Sabre and T'ai Chi Staff practices. Just as the empty-hand forms do, Sword, Sabre, and Staff have their own distinct terms for the Thirteen Postures.

T'ai Chi is all about efficiency of movement, and the Eight Hands are disciplines to that end concerning hand movements. Just as with the waist, the Eight Directions are meticulously maneuvered and positioned to prevent extraneous movement.

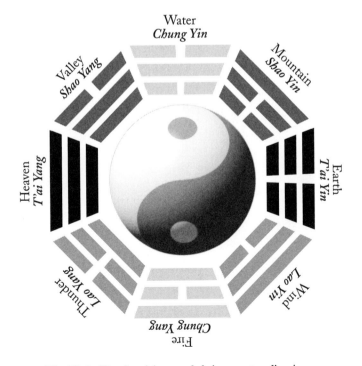

The Eight Hand positions and their corresponding images

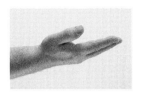

T'ai Yang—*Heaven*

Palm faces upward.

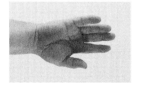

T'ai Yin—*Earth*

Palm faces downward.

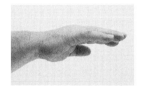

Shao Yang—*Valley*

Palm faces down or diagonally upward.

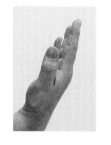

Shao Yin—*Mountain*

Palm faces the body, with fingers pointed diagonally upward.

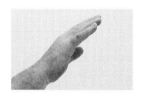

Chung Yang—*Fire*

Palm faces outward.

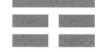

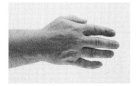

Chung Yin—*Water*

Palm faces inward.

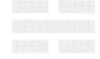

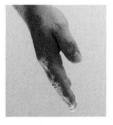

Lao Yang—*Thunder*

Palm faces outward, with fingers pointed downward.

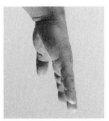

Lao Yin—*Wind*

Palm faces back, with fingers pointed downward.

Hand Variations

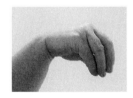

Crane's Beak Hand as used in the Single Whip Posture is a variation of *Shao Yang*.

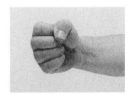

Fist as used in the Deflect, Parry, and Punch Posture is a variation of *Chung Yin*.

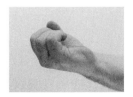

Fist as used in Chop with Fist is a variation of *Shao Yin*.

The Before Heaven 16-Posture Form
Arrangement Charts (circular, square, and linear)

As stated earlier, both the three-lined and six-lined images are to be arranged and viewed in three manners. The I Ching states, "Heaven is seen in the circular, Earth in squareness, and Man in straightness." These charts then provide the reader with both the logic and correctness indicated by the I Ching for the Before Heaven 16-Posture I Ching T'ai Chi arrangement.

CIRCULAR CHART OF THE SIXTEEN POSTURES
(Heaven)

Wu Chi *Position*

Yang *Postures—1 to 8*
Before Heaven Sequence

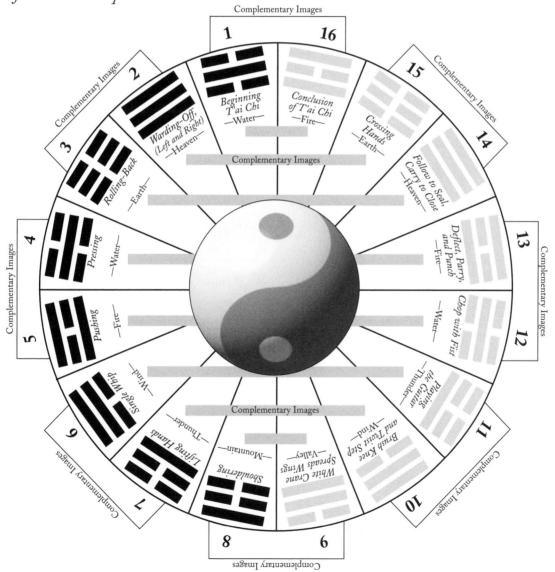

Complementary Images

1   16

2

3

4

5

6

7

8   6

9

10

11

12

13

14

15

Complementary Images

Beginning T'ai Chi —Water—

Conclusion of T'ai Chi —Fire—

Crossing Hands —Earth—

Warding-Off, (Left and Right) —Heaven—

Rolling-Back —Earth—

Pressing —Water—

Pushing —Fire—

Single Whip —Wind—

Lifting Hands —Thunder—

Shouldering —Mountain—

White Crane Spreads Wings —Valley—

Brush Knee and Twist Step —Wind—

Playing the Guitar —Thunder—

Chop with Fist —Water—

Deflect, Parry, and Punch —Fire—

Follow to Seal, Carry to Close —Heaven—

Yin *Postures—9 to 16*
After Heaven Sequence

SQUARE CHART OF THE SIXTEEN POSTURES
(Earth)

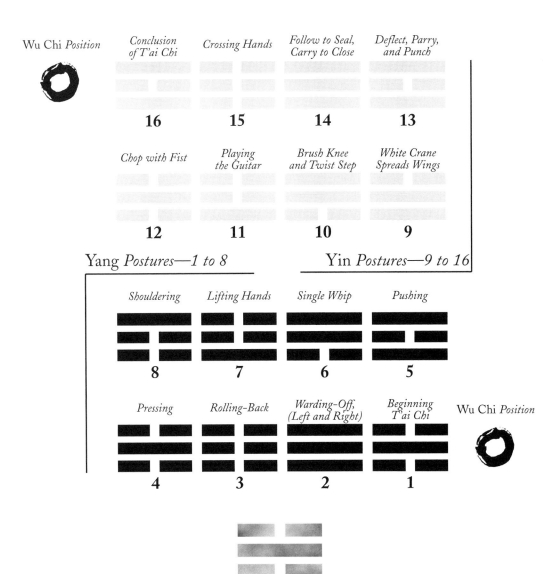

Fire

Wu Chi *Position*	*Conclusion of T'ai Chi*	*Crossing Hands*	*Follow to Seal, Carry to Close*	*Deflect, Parry, and Punch*
	16	**15**	**14**	**13**

Chop with Fist	*Playing the Guitar*	*Brush Knee and Twist Step*	*White Crane Spreads Wings*
12	**11**	**10**	**9**

Yang *Postures—1 to 8*   Yin *Postures—9 to 16*

Shouldering	*Lifting Hands*	*Single Whip*	*Pushing*
8	**7**	**6**	**5**

Pressing	*Rolling-Back*	*Warding-Off, (Left and Right)*	*Beginning T'ai Chi*	Wu Chi *Position*
4	**3**	**2**	**1**	

Water

LINEAR CHART OF THE SIXTEEN POSTURES
(Man)

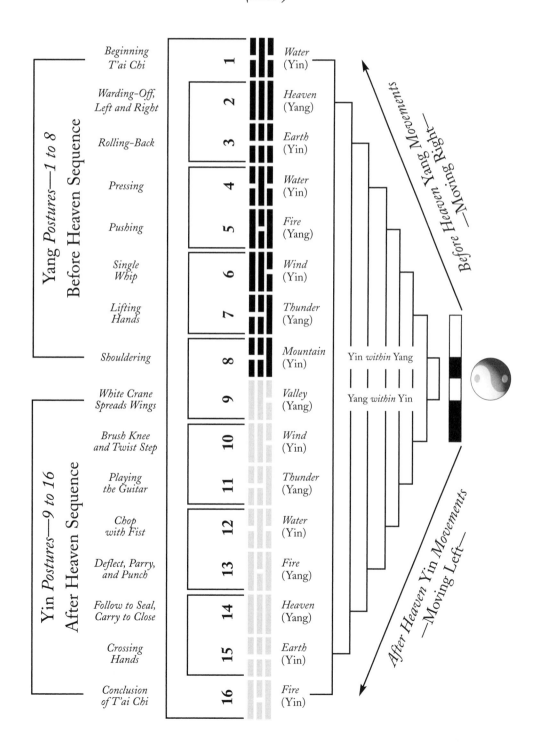

Yang Postures—1 to 8
Before Heaven Sequence

Beginning T'ai Chi	1 — Water (Yin)
Warding-Off, Left and Right	2 — Heaven (Yang)
Rolling-Back	3 — Earth (Yin)
Pressing	4 — Water (Yin)
Pushing	5 — Fire (Yang)
Single Whip	6 — Wind (Yin)
Lifting Hands	7 — Thunder (Yang)
Shouldering	8 — Mountain (Yin)

Yin Postures—9 to 16
After Heaven Sequence

White Crane Spreads Wings	9 — Valley (Yang)
Brush Knee and Twist Step	10 — Wind (Yin)
Playing the Guitar	11 — Thunder (Yang)
Chop with Fist	12 — Water (Yin)
Deflect, Parry, and Punch	13 — Fire (Yang)
Follow to Seal, Carry to Close	14 — Heaven (Yang)
Crossing Hands	15 — Earth (Yin)
Conclusion of T'ai Chi	16 — Fire (Yin)

Before Heaven Yang Movements— —Moving Right

After Heaven Yin Movements— —Moving Left

Yin *within* Yang

Yang *within* Yin

THE BEFORE HEAVEN 16-POSTURE I CHING T'AI CHI FORM

(Hsien T'ien T'ai Chi)

16-Posture T'ai Chi According to the Interaction of the Eight (Trigram) Images

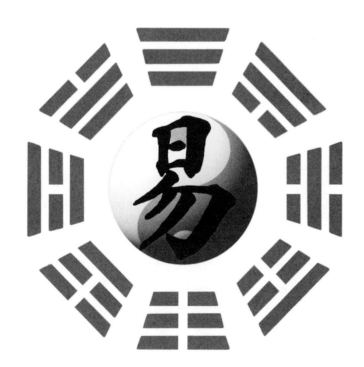

Overview of the Posture Instructional Information

Photographs are provided for each movement of each posture of the Before Heaven Form, along with the following key information.

The first line under the heading for each movement includes the direction the body is to be facing after finishing the movement and indicates whether to inhale or exhale. The direction of the body incorporates the function of the T'ai Chi Waist, which is principled upon the changing movements of the T'ai Chi symbol. In order to comply with the principle of the "square within a circle," the waist turns directly to one of the Eight Directions. This principle is of utmost importance, otherwise the waist will cause the body to either overextend or lose its practical function, like the axle of a wheel, altogether, in which case the eyes cannot match the movements of the waist, or the waist develops no energy. Instructions on whether to inhale or exhale represent the aspects of *yin* and *yang* and of Opening and Closing. Breathing should be natural, not forced. Simply put your attention in the lower abdomen and the breath will follow this intention. The action of the breath should be like a bellows, opening and closing. The postures themselves will induce the breathing, so as you become more proficient in the movements, less and less attention will be focused on the breathing.

The second line of instruction names which of the Five Activities (Advancing, Withdrawing, Looking-Left, Gazing-Right, or Fixed-Rooting) is being used and which of the Five Operations (Rise, Shift, Sink, Turn, or Step) the movements incorporate. (See page 108 for an explanation of the Five Operations).

The third line states which of the Ten T'ai Chi Stances is being applied in the movement—(1) Riding a Horse, (2) Bow and Arrow, (3) Seated Tiger, (4) Seven-Star, (5) Climbing a Mountain, (6) Golden Rooster, (7) Eight Shape, (8) Twisting Dragon, (9) Crawling Snake, or (10) Immortal. In these ten stances the first stance signifies the neutral position of Fixed-Rooting and the remaining nine stances correlate to the Nine Palaces. (See pages 110–120 for explanations on the Ten T'ai Chi Stances.)

The fourth line tells which of the Eight Hand Positions is being used during the movement—(1) *T'ai Yang*, (2) *T'ai Yin*, (3) *Chung Yang*, (4) *Chung Yin*, (5) *Shao Yang*, (6) *Shao Yin*, (7) *Lao Yang*, or (8) *Lao Yin*. (See pages 121–123 for explanations on the Eight Hands.)

Then comes a brief paragraph or two describing how to perform the particular movement cited in the posture.

Following the instructional text for each posture comes a section on the "Images" (the four calculated and related images of the posture), which explains the I Ching meaning of all four images, as well as their implications for T'ai Chi. (See also the Four Arrangements of the Eight Diagrams charts in the section on the Eight Gates).

Before Heaven Image describes the meaning of each line of the image in relation to the posture and at what point in the movement the technique or application is being expressed.

Complementary Image describes the I Ching meaning of the two complements in relation to one another and explains the natural course of action when the Before Heaven and After Heaven techniques fail.

Eight Gates Image describes the best entrance and opportunity for applying its indicated technique and where in the movements of the posture it can be applied.

After Heaven Image describes the I Ching meaning of the Before Heaven and After Heaven images in relation to one another, where the technique of the After Heaven image is applied in the movements, and how each technique creates the opportunity for all other techniques.

Finally, presented under the heading of "Philosophy" are selected statements from the I Ching, *Tao Te Ching*, and the *T'ai Chi Classics* that relate to the posture at hand.

The combination of all these aspects provides an entirely new perspective on T'ai Chi theory, practice, and application. Each of these aspects and correlations is provided within each posture so that the reader may see how all of them function and apply to every movement and posture of T'ai Chi.

First Eight Postures

YANG BEFORE HEAVEN SEQUENCE

Wu Chi Position

FIRST POSTURE	*Beginning T'ai Chi*	*Water* (Yang)
SECOND POSTURE	*Warding-Off, Left Style, Part One* *Right Style, Part Two*	*Heaven* (Yang)
THIRD POSTURE	*Rolling-Back*	*Earth* (Yang)
FOURTH POSTURE	*Pressing*	*Water* (Yang)
FIFTH POSTURE	*Pushing*	*Fire* (Yang)
SIXTH POSTURE	*Single Whip*	*Wind* (Yang)
SEVENTH POSTURE	*Lifting Hands*	*Thunder* (Yang)
EIGHTH POSTURE	*Shouldering*	*Mountain* (Yin *within* Yang)

Wu Chi Position

Wu Chi Shih

Stand erect with the feet positioned at shoulder's width distance apart in a Seated Horse Stance. Make sure the toes are pointed directly ahead (so the toes are then turned slightly inward). In the *Wu Chi* posture for the 16-Posture Form the hands are held in the *Lao Yin* position, but in the After Heaven 64-Posture Form they are held along the sides of the body.

Suspend the head, gaze levelly, place the tongue against the palate, and focus the attention into the *tan-t'ien*. When the breath is slowed and maintained deeply in the lower abdomen, and the mind is tranquil, then the T'ai Chi movements of separating *yin* and *yang* can begin.

Perform at least three complete breaths before moving on to the first posture.

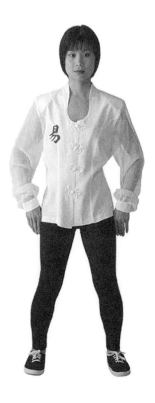

IMAGE

 Wu Chi (the Illimitable) is the state in which *yin* and *yang* have not yet separated. There is no movement, no change, no thought. All is in a state of perfect tranquillity.

Chou Tun-i, the neo-Confucian Sung-dynasty philosopher, was the first to coin this term, which has become a standard Taoist depiction for the condition of the universe, the illimitable state of Tao, before Heaven and Earth came into existence.

The image of *Wu Chi* is always the circle because it has no beginning and no end, making it infinite. T'ai Chi is then the image of the circle being broken and separated into *yin* and *yang* movement.

PHILOSOPHY

I Ching

One senses that the body no longer exists. The wise man's thoughts do not go beyond this position.

Tao Te Ching

The Tao proceeds only through natural movement. From the Tao comes the One, from the One comes Two, from Two comes Three, and from Three comes the Ten-Thousand Things.

T'ai Chi Ch'uan Classics

T'ai Chi is born of *Wu Chi*, the mother of *yin* and *yang*. In motion they separate; in tranquillity they unite.

Beginning T'ai Chi

T'ai Chi Ch'i Shih

Before Heaven Image of K'an—Water (Pressing)

FIRST POSTURE

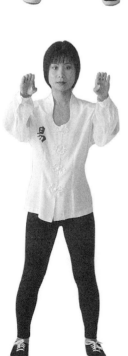

1st Movement
North—*Inhale*
Rise
Seated Horse
Both Hands, *Lao Yin*
Inhale as you let the hands float upward with fingertips pointing down, the knuckles pointing to the front, and the arms held at shoulder height.

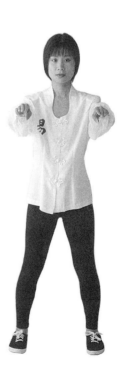

2nd Movement
North—*Exhale*
Sink
Seated Horse
Both Hands, *T'ai Yin*
Exhale as the fingers are extended to the front with the arms still held at shoulder height.

3rd Movement
North—*Inhale*
Rise
Seated Horse
Both Hands, *Shao Yang*
Inhale as the hands float upward to a 45-degree angle.

4th Movement
North—*Exhale*
Sink
Seated Horse
Both Hands, *T'ai Yin*
Exhale and lower the elbows
so that the fingertips are out from
the bottom of the chest.

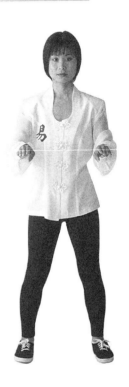

5th Movement
North—*Inhale*
Rise
Seated Horse
Both Hands, *Lao Yin*
Inhale as the hands float down
with the palms facing the
front of the thighs.

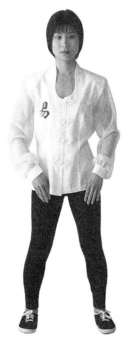

6th Movement
North—*Exhale*
Sink
Seated Horse
Both Hands, *Lao Yin*
Exhale as the elbows are pressed forward
and the hands are brought to the hips,
palms facing behind.

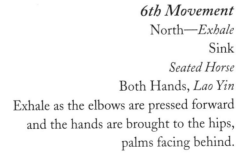
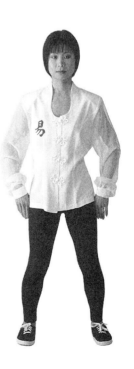

IMGES

Before Heaven Image—Water/Pressing

Yin is in the arms and palms. They float as if in water with the Mind-Intent. *Yang* is in the abdomen, where the blood and *ch'i* are stimulated. *Yin* is seen in the feet and legs, rising and sinking as if in water. Pressing is symbolic here, showing that the breath and *ch'i* are being sunk into the *tan-t'ien.*

Complementary Image—Fire/Pushing

When Fire is below Water, the water can then be made to move. When the *ch'i* stimulates the *ching,* the internal energies can be made to move. In this posture, Water is still beneath Fire, but through the movements of the remaining postures the *ch'i* will sink into the *tan-t'ien,* bringing Fire beneath Water. This is the first and most important process of internal cultivation. If both Pressing and Elbowing fail, the most natural course is to use Pushing, which can be initiated in the transition of the 3rd and 4th movements.

Eight Gates Image—Thunder/Splitting

The Beginning T'ai Chi Posture is like a vibration (Thunder) coming up from the Earth to move and stimulate the Fire and Water into their correct positions. Water is pressed below Fire and Fire is being pushed up from the Earth by Thunder (the movements). The best stimulus for Water is to first use Thunder to stimulate it. In the *T'ai Chi Ch'uan Treatise,* when it says "the energy (Thunder) is rooted in the feet (Earth), developed in the legs, directed by the waist (Water), and appears in the hands and fingers (Fire)," it is being very descriptive of these images.

After Heaven Image—Valley/Elbowing

Water cannot be visible nor can it exist without Valley, through which it flows and in which it is collected. Pressing is supported by and rests upon the actions of Elbowing. If Pressing is interrupted, then Elbowing can be initiated in the 2nd and 3rd movements.

PHILOSOPHY

I Ching

The movement of Heaven is full of strength; the wise man strengthens himself unceasingly.

Tao Te Ching

When the mind rests in the state of nothingness, look at the internal aspects; when the mind produces an inner state, look at the external aspects.

T'ai Chi Ch'uan Classics

When using the techniques of Adhering, Joining, Sticking, and Following with no resistance and with no letting go in Sensing-Hands practice, we look at the internal aspects of Neutralizing; when Issuing energy to attack, we look at the external aspects.

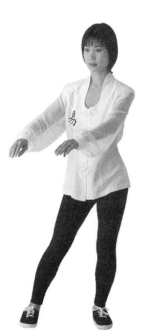

Warding-Off, Left Style

Tso P'eng

Before Heaven Image of Ch'ien—Heaven *(Warding-Off)*

SECOND POSTURE (PART ONE)

1st Movement
Northeast—*Inhale*
Gazing-Right—Shift, Sink, Turn
Riding a Horse, Left
Both Hands, *T'ai Yin*
Inhale as you shift all the weight into the left leg and begin turning the waist and body to face NE. The hands float upward equally and in line to a 45-degree angle from the level of the shoulders.

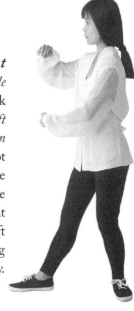

2nd Movement
East—*Exhale*
Gazing-Right—Rise, Turn, Sink
Seven Star, Left
L Hand, *T'ai Yang*—R Hand, *T'ai Yin*
Exhale as you continue turning right and to the E. The right-foot toes are held off the ground, with only the heel touching until the posture is completed and the foot is placed flat onto the ground. The hands simultaneously float upward as the waist turns. The right hand and arm float up to neck level, with palm facing down; the left hand floats up to only lower abdomen level, with palm facing upward. The hands appear to be holding a ball out from the body.

3rd Movement
East—*Inhale*
Advancing—Rise, Shift, Sink
Bow and Arrow, Right
L Hand, *T'ai Yang*—R Hand, *T'ai Yin*
With the right foot flat, inhale as you shift all your weight into the right leg. The hands and arms remain in the same position.

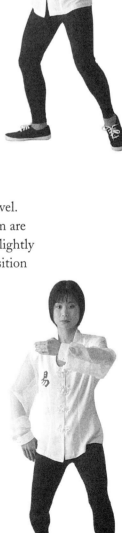

4th Movement

Northeast—*Exhale*
Looking-Left—Rise, Turn, Sink
Seated Tiger, Right
L Hand, *T'ai Yang*—R Hand, *T'ai Yin*

Exhale as you begin turning the waist and body to the left and NE corner by rising a little, then turning and finally sinking. When turning, the left-foot heel is raised off the ground, with only the toes touching. The hands do not move from their previous position during this movement.

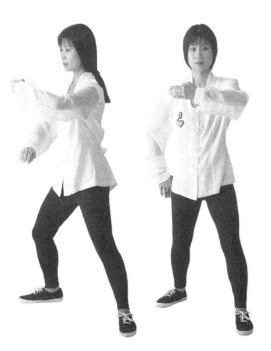

5th Movement

North—*Inhale*
Advancing—Sink, Step, Shift
Looking-Left—Rise, Turn
Bow and Arrow, Left
L Hand, *Chung Yin*—R Hand, *Lao Yin*

Inhale as you simultaneously step directly forward with the left foot (onto the heel first before placing the foot flat) while bringing the left hand and arm up to shoulder level. Raise the left arm upward until the hand and arm are on line with the upper chest area, with the arm slightly bowed as if holding a ball until it reaches the position of being along the right side of the waist and the fingers pointing outward. The waist and body at this point are still facing NE.

Next, shift the weight into the left leg and pick up the right toes. Pivoting on the heel, turn the waist to the left. The toes of the right foot are turned to point to the NE, where the foot is then placed flat.

6th Movement

North—*Exhale*
Fixed-Rooting—Sink
Bow and Arrow, Left
L Hand, *Chung Yin*—R Hand, *Lao Yin*

Exhale as you sink the entire body downward so that approximately 70 percent of the weight is in the forward (left) leg and 30 percent in the rear leg.

IMAGES

 Before Heaven Image—Heaven/Warding-Off, **Left Style** *Yang* **is in the left forearm.**

Yang is in left side of the trunk of the body.

Yang is in the front, left foot and leg.

Warding-Off, Left Style occurs in the transitions of the 4th and 5th movements.

Complementary Image—Earth/Rolling-Back

Heaven must precede and depend on Earth and Fire for expression. Warding-Off must precede and depend on Rolling-Back.

If both Warding-Off and Pushing fail, the most natural course is to use Rolling-Back, which can be initiated in the transitions of the 1st, 2nd, and 5th movements.

Eight Gates Image—Water/Pressing

The best stimulus for applying Warding-Off is to first use Pressing. Water and Fire are the two auspicious servants of Heaven and Earth. Water serves and collects on Earth, and Fire serves to give brilliance to Heaven. When Warding-Off or Rolling-Back fails, Pressing or Pushing can be used. Pressing aids Rolling-Back, and Pushing aids Warding-Off.

After Heaven Image—Fire/Pushing

Just as Heaven is revealed by light (Fire), within Warding-Off there is Pushing, and it can be initiated either in the transitions of the 3rd or 5th movements. The postures Warding-Off (Left and Right), Rolling-Back, Pressing, and Pushing in the 64-Posture I Ching T'ai Chi Form are called, collectively, Grasping the Bird's Tail—which begins with Warding-Off and concludes with Pushing.

PHILOSOPHY

I Ching

With utmost humility the wise man receives people. Tranquillity always invites good results.

Tao Te Ching

Nothingness and something create each other; back and front follow each other.

T'ai Chi Ch'uan Classics

When the opponent places pressure on your left side, it should be empty; the same is true for your right side. When Advancing, the opponent feels the distance is incredibly long. When Withdrawing, he feels the distance is exasperatingly short.

Warding-Off, Right Style

Yu P'eng

SECOND POSTURE (PART TWO)*

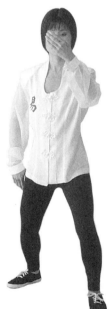

1st Movement

North—*Inhale*

Advancing—Rise, Sink

Bow and Arrow, Left

L Hand, *Shao Yin*—R Hand, *Lao Yin*

Inhale as you rise up, picking up the rear (right) heel as you do so. Simultaneously, drop the left elbow to hang at a 45-degree angle relative to the level of the shoulder, while bringing the left palm over to face directly in front of the nose. Slightly seat the entire body.

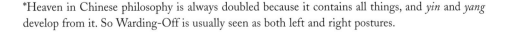

2nd Movement

Northeast—*Exhale*

Gazing-Right—Rise, Turn, Sink

Seated Tiger, Left

L Hand, *T'ai Yin*—R Hand, *T'ai Yang*

Exhale as you turn the waist and body to the right to face NE while dropping the left elbow so that the hand is held at lower-neck level with the palm facing diagonally downward to the NE. The right hand simultaneously floats upward to the lower abdomen level. While turning the body, with the right heel off the ground, pivot the foot right until the toes point E. Seat the entire body slightly after turning right to the NE.

---

*Heaven in Chinese philosophy is always doubled because it contains all things, and *yin* and *yang* develop from it. So Warding-Off is usually seen as both left and right postures.

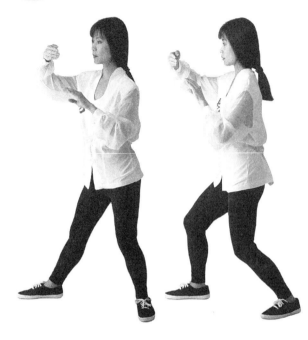

3rd Movement

East—*Inhale*
Advancing—Sink, Step, Shift
Gazing-Right—Rise, Turn
Bow and Arrow, Right
L Hand, *Shao Yang*—R Hand, *Chung Yin*

Inhale as you step forward and out with the right foot onto the heel, then placing the foot flat. Simultaneously bring the right hand up so that the palm faces the nose. The waist and body at this point are still facing NE.

Next, shift the weight into the right leg, then pick up the left toes and turn the waist and body right to face E. The toes of the left foot are turned right to point to the NE, with the entire foot then being placed down.

The left hand and arm turn with the body, so that the fingers end about 6 inches below and behind the right palm, fingers pointing diagonally upward.

4th Movement

East—*Exhale*
Fixed-Rooting—Sink
Bow and Arrow, Right
L Hand, *Shao Yang*—R Hand, *Chung Yin*

Exhale as you sink the entire body downward so that approximately 70 percent of the weight is in the forward (right) leg and 30 percent in the left.

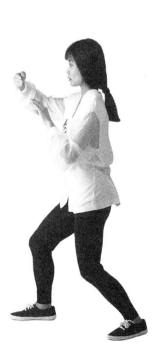

IMAGES

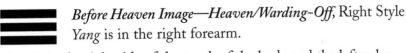 *Before Heaven Image—Heaven/Warding-Off,* Right Style
Yang is in the right forearm.

Yang is in the right side of the trunk of the body and the left palm.

Yang is in the right, forward leg and foot.

Warding-Off, Right Style occurs in the transitions of the 2nd and 3rd movements.

Complementary Image—Earth/Rolling-Back

Heaven must precede and depend on Earth, and on Fire for expression. Warding-Off precedes Rolling-Back, and Pushing follows. If both Warding-Off and Pushing fail, the most natural course is in Rolling-Back. Rolling-Back can be initiated in the transitions of the 1st, 3rd, and 4th movements.

Eight Gates Image—Water/Pressing

The best stimulus for applying Warding-Off is when the opponent uses Pressing. Water and Fire are the two auspicious servants of Heaven and Earth. Water serves and collects on the Earth, and Fire serves to give brilliance to Heaven. When Warding-Off or Rolling-Back fails, Pressing or Pushing can be used. Pressing aids Rolling-Back, and Pushing aids Warding-Off.

After Heaven Image—Fire/Pushing

Just as Heaven is revealed by light (Fire), within Warding-Off there is Pushing, and it can be initiated in the transitions of the 3rd movement.

PHILOSOPHY
(SAME AS WARDING-OFF, LEFT STYLE)

I Ching

With utmost humility the wise man receives people. Tranquillity always invites good results.

Tao Te Ching

Nothingness and something create each other; back and front follow each other.

T'ai Chi Ch'uan Classics

When the opponent places pressure on your left side, it should be empty; the same is true for your right side. When Advancing, the opponent feels the distance is incredibly long. When Withdrawing, he feels the distance is exasperatingly short.

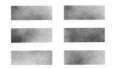

Rolling-Back

Lü

Before Heaven Image of K'un—Earth *(Rolling-Back)*

THIRD POSTURE

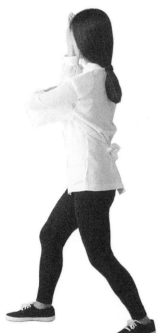

1st Movement

East—*Inhale*

Gazing-Right—Rise, Turn, Sink

Bow and Arrow, Right

L Hand, *Chung Yin*—R Hand, *Shao Yin*

Inhale as you turn your waist and body to the right to the SE
corner. Simultaneously bring your right-hand fingers to point
upward while keeping the same bend in the elbow from
the previous posture. At the same time, move the left hand
across at chest level and place the fingertips on the
inner part of the right elbow.

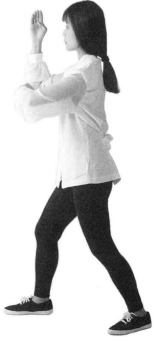

2nd Movement

East—*Exhale*

Looking-Left—Rise, Turn, Sink

Bow and Arrow, Right

L Hand, *Chung Yin*—R Hand, *Shao Yin*

Exhale as you turn the waist and body back
to the left to face E, keeping the arms in the same
position as they move with the body.

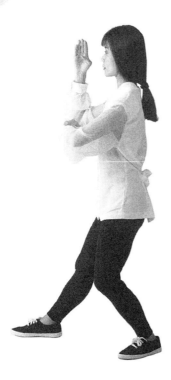

3rd Movement

East—*Inhale*

Withdrawing—Rise, Shift, Sink

Climbing a Mountain, Left

L Hand, *Chung Yin*—R Hand, *Shao Yin*

Inhale as you shift and sink back into the rear (left) leg. As you do so, lower the elbows of the arms while maintaining the same position so that the left forearm is parallel to the middle abdomen area.

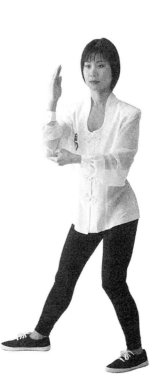

4th Movement

Northeast—*Exhale*

Looking-Left, Fixed-Rooting—Turn, Sink

Climbing a Mountain, Left

L Hand, *T'ai Yang*—R Hand, *Shao Yin*

Exhale as you turn your waist and body to the left to the NE. Simultaneously drop the left elbow so that the left palm is turned up, with fingertips still adhering to the inner right elbow.

IMAGES

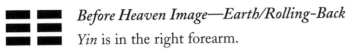

Before Heaven Image—Earth/Rolling-Back

Yin is in the right forearm.

Yin is in the left side of the body.

Yin is in the right, front foot.

Rolling-Back occurs in the 1st and 4th movements. Rolling-Back is the most important posture and energy in all of T'ai Chi; mastering it in all its aspects means mastering half of T'ai Chi.

Complementary Image—Heaven/Warding-Off

Earth looks to Heaven for completion and to Water for nourishment. Rolling-Back comes from Warding-Off and moves into Pressing. When Rolling-Back and Pressing fail, the most natural course is to use Warding-Off, which can be initiated in the 1st and 3rd movements.

Eight Gates Image—Fire/Pushing

The best stimulus for applying Rolling-Back is when the opponent uses Pushing. Water and Fire are the two auspicious servants of Heaven and Earth. Water serves Earth, and Fire serves Heaven. When Rolling-Back or Warding-Off fails, Pressing or Pushing can be used. Pressing aids Rolling-Back, and Pushing aids Warding-Off.

After Heaven Image—Water/Pressing

Earth is revealed by and depends on Water. Within Rolling-Back there is Pressing, and it can be initiated in the 2nd movement and following the 4th movement.

PHILOSOPHY

I Ching

The Earth's condition is to be receptive. The greatness of the wise man's character is to endure everything.

Tao Te Ching

The entire universe is like a bellows; it is hollow, yet it is inexhaustible. The more it works, the more comes out of it.

T'ai Chi Ch'uan Classics

The energy appears relaxed, but is not empty. The more pressure you put on me, the more reaction force you will receive.

Pressing

Chi

Before Heaven Image of K'an—*Water (Pressing)*

FOURTH POSTURE

1st Movement
North—*Inhale*
Looking-Left—Rise, Turn, Sink
Climbing a Mountain, Left
L Hand, *T'ai Yang*—R Hand, *Shao Yin*
Inhale as you turn your waist and body to the left to the N, bringing the left hand back with palm facing up and the right hand staying in its previous position.

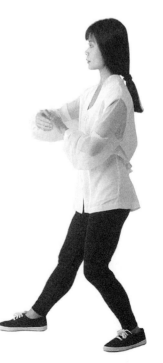

2nd Movement
East—*Exhale*
Gazing-Right—Rise, Turn, Sink
Climbing a Mountain, Left
L Hand, *Shao Yang*—R Hand, *Chung Yin*
Exhale as you turn your waist and body back to the right to face E. Lower the right forearm so that it is held levelly in front of the lower abdomen with the palm facing the body, while bringing the left-hand fingertips onto the inner right wrist.

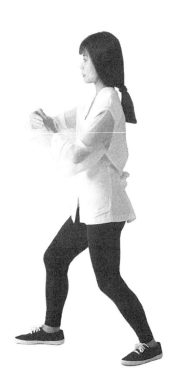

3rd Movement

East—*Inhale*

Advancing, Looking-Left—Rise, Turn, Shift

Gazing-Right—Turn, Sink

Bow and Arrow, Right

L Hand, *Shao Yang*—R Hand, *Chung Yin*

Inhale as you make a slight turning gesture to the left while shifting your weight forward. After shifting into the forward leg, turn the body back to the right and front while sinking and rerooting into the right leg. Keep the arms in the same position when shifting and sinking.

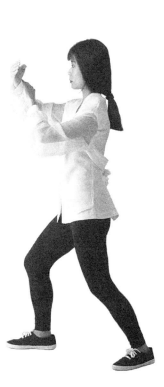

4th Movement

East—*Exhale*

Advancing—Rise

Fixed-Rooting—Sink

Bow and Arrow, Right

L Hand, *Shao Yang*—R Hand, **Chung Yin**

Exhale as you rise off your rear leg (keeping the feet flat on the ground) and bring the arms slightly upward and out, slightly dropping both elbows. Last, sink the entire body downward so that approximately 70 percent of the weight is in the right leg and 30 percent in the rear (left) leg.

IMAGES

 Before Heaven Image—Water/Pressing

Yin is in the right forearm.

Yang is in the left, rear hand.

Yin is in the rear, left leg and foot.

Pressing occurs in the transitions of the 3rd and 4th movements. Pressing shows a force that conceals strength, *yang*. Thus the left hand (the actual Pressing hand) is enveloped within the *yin* rear (left) leg and the *yin* front (right) arm. Although the substance of water feels soft and appears insubstantial, within it lies a great strength.

Complementary Image—Fire/Pushing

Water seeks the low places of the Valley and Fire seeks to rise upward from the Valley. Pressing should retain the intent of Elbowing but rely on Pushing. If no opportunity arises for Pressing or Elbowing, Pushing is then the natural response and can be initiated in the 3rd movement.

Eight Gates Image—Thunder/Splitting

The best stimulus for applying Pressing is when the opponent uses Splitting. Thunder and Valley rely on the support of Water and Fire. Valley serves to store Water, and Thunder serves to stimulate Fire. When Pressing and Pushing fail, Elbowing or Splitting can be used. Elbowing aids Pressing, and Splitting aids Pushing.

After Heaven Image—Valley/Elbowing

Water fills the low places, Valleys. Within Pressing there is Elbowing, and it can be initiated in the transitions of either the 1st and 2nd movements or in the 3rd and 4th movements. Elbowing is Folding-Up Energy. If the wrist is seized, the elbow strikes. If the elbow is seized, the shoulder strikes. If the shoulder is seized, the head strikes. Folding-up is like filling the empty spaces. This comes from the story given earlier of Chang San-feng watching the snake's responses to the attacks and strikes of the bird.

PHILOSOPHY

I Ching

The wise man carefully distinguishes the position of things and puts them in their proper place.

Tao Te Ching

He chooses to be last and so becomes first. Reckons himself outside and finds himself safe and secure. In all the world nothing is stronger than water.

T'ai Chi Ch'uan Classics

If your opponent does not move, you do not move; at his slightest stir you have already anticipated it and move beforehand. If you go your own way, your movements will be clumsy. If you give yourself up and follow others, your movements will be light and alert.

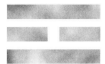

Pushing

An

Before Heaven Image of Li—*Fire (Pushing)*

FIFTH POSTURE

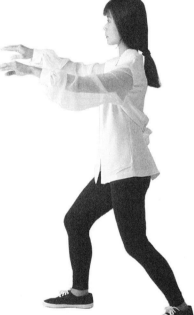

1st Movement
East—*Inhale*
Advancing—Rise, Sink
Bow and Arrow, Right
Both Hands, *T'ai Yin*
Inhale as you separate both hands in front of the body, as if wiping something off the back of the right hand with the left palm, bringing them to a shoulders' width distance apart. Rise and sink slightly with this movement.

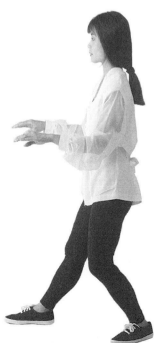

2nd Movement
East—*Exhale*
Withdrawing, Looking-Left—
Rise, Turn, Shift, Sink
Climbing a Mountain, Left
Both Hands, *T'ai Yin*
Exhale as you make a slight turning gesture while shifting back and sinking into the rear (left) leg. Simultaneously, drop both elbows and bring the forearms and palms to a parallel position at midabdomen level.

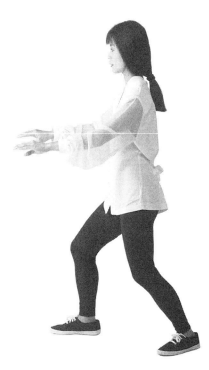

3rd Movement

East—*Inhale*
Advancing—Rise, Shift, Sink
Bow and Arrow, Right
Both Hands, *T'ai Yin*
Inhale as you shift your weight back into the right leg, keeping the arms and hands in the same position.

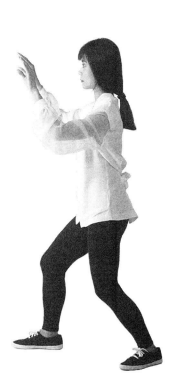

4th Movement

East—*Exhale*
Advancing—Rise
Fixed-Rooting—Sink
Bow and Arrow, Right
Both Hands, *Shao Yang*
Exhale as you rise off your rear leg (keeping the feet flat on the ground) while bringing the arms upward and out, slightly dropping the elbows. Keep the palms facing out. Last, sink the body downward so that approximately 70 percent of the weight is in the forward leg and 30 percent in the rear.

IMAGES

 Before Heaven Image—Fire/Pushing

Yang is in the left palm.

Yin is in the right hand and arm.

Yang is in the right front leg.

Pushing occurs in the transitions of the 3rd and 4th movements. Pushing must come from the rear foot, just as a fire rises from its fuel—this is the bottom *yang* line. The shoulders and arms must be relaxed, without using physical strength—this is the middle *yin* line. The Push must be expressed through the hands, like the tip of a whip, or the tip of a flame—this is the top *yang* line.

Complementary Image—Water/Pressing

Fire is generated by Thunder, and Thunder stimulates the rain (Water). Pushing must retain the intent of Splitting but rely on Pressing. If no opportunity arises for Pushing or Splitting, Pressing is then the natural response and can be initiated in the 2nd movement.

Eight Gates Image—Valley/Elbowing

The best stimulus for applying Pushing is when the opponent uses Elbowing. Thunder and Valley rely on the support of Fire and Water. Thunder serves to stimulate Fire, and Valley serves to store Water. When Pushing and Pressing fail, Splitting or Elbowing can be used. Splitting aids Pushing, and Elbowing aids Pressing.

After Heaven Image—Thunder/Splitting

Fire is created by Thunder. Within Pushing there is Splitting, and it can be initiated in either the 1st or 2nd movement. Pushing is entirely generated from the issuance of *chin* (intrinsic energy, symbolized by Thunder). Pushing is like a flame rising quickly and then receding, destroying everything in its path.

PHILOSOPHY

I Ching

The city might be moved, but not the well. It neither overflows nor runs dry.

Tao Te Ching

The Tao is imperceptible and its usefulness is limitless.

T'ai Chi Ch'uan Classics

Appearing relaxed, but not empty; ready to expand, but not yet expanding.

Single Whip

Tan Pien

Before Heaven Image of **Sun**—*Wind (Pulling)*

SIXTH POSTURE

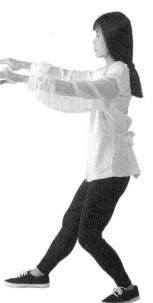

1st Movement

East—*Inhale*

Withdrawing—Rise, Shift, Sink

Climbing a Mountain, Left

Both Hands, *T'ai Yin*

Inhale as you shift your weight back into the left leg. When shifting back, lower the hands to shoulder height while holding the arms and hands parallel to the ground. Keep the body facing E.

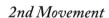

2nd Movement

North—*Exhale*

Looking-Left—Rise, Turn, Sink

Eight Shape, Left

Both Hands, *T'ai Yin*

Exhale as you turn the entire waist, right toes, and body to the left to face N, keeping the arms in the same position.

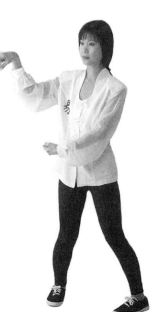

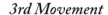

3rd Movement

Northeast—*Inhale*

Gazing-Right—Shift, Turn, Sink

Eight Shape, Right

L Hand, *T'ai Yang*—R Hand, *Shao Yang**

Inhale as you shift to the right leg, turn your waist to face NE, and sink your weight. Simultaneously, draw the left hand down, palm up, to the front of the lower abdomen; drop the right elbow and form a hook with the five fingers, of the hand hand. The knuckles face left the NE corner.

4th Movement

Northwest—*Exhale*
Looking-Left—Rise, Turn, Sink
Seated Tiger, Right
L Hand, *T'ai Yang*—R Hand, *Shao Yang**
Exhale as you rise up, pick the left heel
off the ground, and turn right to face NW.
While doing so, extend the right-hand
hook out toward the N and pivot the
left toes so that they point to
the right, the NW corner.

5th Movement

West—*Inhale*
Advancing—Sink, Step, Shift
Looking-Left—Rise, Turn, Sink
Bow and Arrow, Left
L Hand, *Shao Yin*—R Hand, *Shao Yang**
Inhale as you trace your left-foot toes along
the floor slightly to the back and then out and
forward, placing the heel down first. Simultaneously,
the left hand floats upward, with fingers pointing
upward and with the arm moving in conjunction
with the left leg. The waist and body at this point are still facing NW.
Next, shift the weight into the left leg and then pick up the right toes
and turn the waist and body left to face W. The toes of the right foot
are turned to point to the NW and then placed back onto the floor.

6th Movement

West—*Exhale*
Fixed-Rooting—Sink
Bow and Arrow, Left
L Hand, *Shao Yang*—R Hand, *Shao Yang**
Exhale as you sink the entire body downward so that approximately 70
percent of the weight is in the right leg and 30 percent in the left.
Simultaneously turn the left palm to face outward.

---

* The right-hand fingers are dropped together, like holding a drop of water. This
hand position is called the "Crane's Beak" and is only seen in the Single Whip postures. In the 64-Posture Form it is also seen in the Glide Down Like Snake postures.

IMAGES

 Before Heaven Image—Wind/Pulling

Yang is in the left palm.

Yang is in the forward hip.

Yin is in the rear foot.

Pulling occurs in the 1st and 2nd and in the transitions of the 4th and 5th movements. Single Whip (Pulling) techniques occur in the 2nd, 3rd, 5th, and 6th movements.

Complementary Image—Thunder/Splitting

Wind is generated by the movements of the Earth, and Thunder can activate the Wind. Pulling must retain the intent of Rolling-Back but rely on Splitting. If no opportunity arises for Pulling or Rolling-Back, Splitting is then the natural response and can be initiated in the 2nd, 3rd, and 5th movements.

Eight Gates Image—Mountain/Shouldering

The best stimulus for applying Pulling is when the opponent uses Shouldering. Earth and Mountain rely on the support of Wind and Thunder. Wind disperses things across the Earth, and Thunder moves and creates the Mountain. When Pulling and Splitting fail, Rolling-Back or Shouldering can be used. Rolling-Back aids Pulling, and Shouldering aids Splitting.

After Heaven Image—Earth/Rolling-Back

The Wind blows over the Earth. Within Pulling there is Rolling-Back, and Rolling-Back can be initiated in either the 1st or 2nd movement.

PHILOSOPHY

I Ching

Observe the natural ways of Heaven and Earth in seeking to direct others.

Tao Te Ching

When you maintain your *shen* and *ch'i* within your body, you can achieve perfect harmony. When your *ch'i* is concentrated to the utmost degree of pliancy, you will achieve the pliability of a child.

T'ai Chi Ch'uan Classics

From the most pliable and yielding comes the most powerful and unyielding.

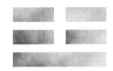

Lifting Hands

T'i Shou

Before Heaven Image of **Chen**—*Thunder (Splitting)*

SEVENTH POSTURE

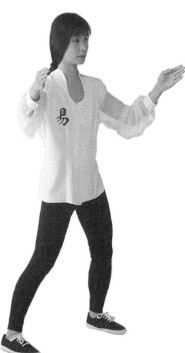

1st Movement
Northwest—*Inhale*
Gazing-Right—Shift, Turn, Shift
Immortal, Left
Both Hands, *Chung Yin*
Inhale as you shift your weight into your right leg, turn in the left foot 20 degrees, and then immediately shift the weight back into the left foot. This shifting back and forth is like a rocking action. Simultaneously, open both hands and turn the palms to face each other.

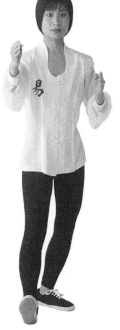

2nd Movement
North—*Exhale*
Gazing-Right—Rise, Turn, Step, Sink
Seven Star, Left
Both Hands, *Chung Yin*
Exhale as you bring the right leg and arm over directly to the N. The right-foot heel is placed on the ground, with toes up. The left-hand palm faces the right elbow.
Seat the waist.

IMAGES

 Before Heaven Image—Thunder/Splitting

Yin is in the left palm.

Yin is in the forward hip.

Yang is in the rear leg.

Lifting Hands (Splitting) occurs in the 2nd movement.

Complementary Image—Wind/Pulling

Thunder and Wind create excitement in nature. Splitting must retain the intent of Shouldering but rely on Pulling. If no opportunity arises for Splitting or Shouldering, Pulling is then the natural response and can be initiated in the 1st movement.

Eight Gates Image—Earth/Rolling-Back

The best stimulus for applying Splitting is when the opponent uses Rolling-Back. Thunder and Wind rely on the support of Mountain and Earth. Thunder serves to move Mountain, and Earth creates and supports the Wind. When Splitting and Pulling fail, Shouldering or Rolling-Back can be used. Shouldering aids Splitting, and Rolling-Back aids Pulling.

After Heaven Image—Mountain/Shouldering

Thunder (shifting and shaking) creates the Mountain. Within Splitting there is Shouldering, and it can be initiated in the transition from the 1st to the 2nd movement.

PHILOSOPHY

I Ching

Water flows unceasingly to the lowest places. The wise man constantly preserves his virtue and practices what he has learned.

Tao Te Ching

The highest form of goodness is like water; in choosing your dwelling, know to keep to the low ground.

T'ai Chi Ch'uan Classics

To detect the defects on an opponent and obtain a superior position, conceal your *ch'i* and *shen* internally and do not expose them externally.

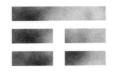

Shouldering

Kao

Before Heaven Image of **Ken**— *Mountain (Shouldering)*

EIGHTH POSTURE

1st Movement
Northwest—*Inhale*
Looking-Left—Rise, Turn
Gazing-Right—Turn, Sink, Step
Climbing a Mountain, Left
Both Hands, *Chung Yin*

Inhale as you pick up your right foot and knee, and turn the waist and body to the left, the NW corner—standing in Golden Rooster, left. Simultaneously, position both hands to be pointing diagonally downward and still shoulders' width apart.

Continue the turning movement to the right, bringing the waist directly back to the N, and bring the right foot forward and to the right, set the foot down by placing the heel down first, and then lowering the entire foot to the ground. Sink the weight into the rear (left) leg. The left hand simultaneously adheres to the inner right elbow; the right hand is lowered so that the palm is facing the lower body.

2nd Movement
North—*Exhale*
Advancing—Rise, Shift
Fixed-Rooting—Sink
Bow and Arrow, Right
Both Hands, *Chung Yin*

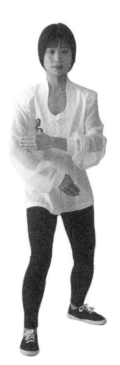

Exhale as you rise off your rear leg, shift the weight forward to the front leg, and then sink the entire body downward so that approximately 70 percent of the weight is in the right leg and 30 percent in the left leg.

IMAGES

 Before Heaven Image—Mountain/Shouldering

Yang is in the right shoulder and arm.

Yin is in the left palm and hip.

Yin is in the rear foot.

Shouldering occurs when shifting into the front leg.

Complementary Image—Valley/Elbowing

The higher the Mountain the deeper the Valley, and thus the greater Heaven appears. Shouldering must retain the intent of Warding-Off but rely on Elbowing. If no opportunity arises for Shouldering or Warding-Off, Elbowing is then the natural response and can be initiated in the 1st movement.

Eight Gates Image—Wind/Pulling

The best stimulus for applying Shouldering is when the opponent uses Elbowing. Heaven and Wind rely on the support of Mountain and Valley. Mountain seeks to reach Heaven, and Valley contains the Wind. When Shouldering and Elbowing fail, Warding-Off or Pulling can be used. Warding-Off aids Shouldering, and Pulling aids Elbowing. The Wind in the Heaven (sky) moves down the Mountain and into the Valley.

After Heaven Image—Heaven/Warding-Off

Heaven brings vastness and greatness to a Mountain. Within Shouldering there is Warding-Off, and it can be initiated in the transition from the 1st to the 2nd movement.

PHILOSOPHY

I Ching

The wise man reduces what is excessive and increases what is deficient. He weighs all things and makes them equal and right.

Tao Te Ching

Things that bend can become whole again; the crooked can become straight.

T'ai Chi Ch'uan Classics

Seek straightness within the curved; this is to put the energy in reserve before releasing it.

Second Eight Postures

YIN AFTER HEAVEN SEQUENCE

NINTH POSTURE	*White Crane Spreads Wings*	*Valley* (Yang *within* Yin)	
TENTH POSTURE	*Brush Knee and Twist Step*	*Wind* (Yin)	
ELEVENTH POSTURE	*Playing the Guitar*	*Thunder* (Yin)	
TWELFTH POSTURE	*Chop with Fist*	*Water* (Yin)	
THIRTEENTH POSTURE	*Deflect, Parry, and Punch*	*Fire* (Yin)	
FOURTEENTH POSTURE	*Follow to Seal, Carry to Close*	*Heaven* (Yin)	
FIFTEENTH POSTURE	*Crossing Hands*	*Earth* (Yin)	
SIXTEENTH POSTURE	*Conclusion of T'ai Chi*	*Fire* (Yin)	

Wu Chi *Position*

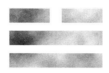

White Crane Spreads Wings

Pai Hao Liang Ch'ih
After Heaven Image of T'ui—*Valley (Elbowing)*

NINTH POSTURE

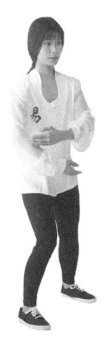

1st Movement
Northwest—*Inhale*
Looking-Left—Shift, Turn, Shift, Sink
Eight Shape, Right
L Hand, *Chung Yin*—R Hand, *T'ai Yang*
Inhale as you shift your weight into the left leg, immediately turn your right
foot inward 20 degrees, and then shift the weight directly back into the
right leg. Simultaneously, bring your left palm to be over the right elbow,
about six inches away; the right palm turns face up. Your waist and
body face NW at this point.

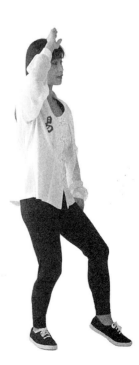

2nd Movement
West—*Exhale*
Looking-Left—Rise, Turn
Fixed-Rooting—Sink
Seated Tiger, Right
L Hand, *Lao Yin*—R Hand, *Chung Yang*
Exhale as you turn your waist to the left to face W and bring the
left foot over, with only the toes touching the ground, to be directly out
from the right heel. Simultaneously bring the left hand over to the left
side of the body, and bring the right upward so that it ends above
the forehead with palm facing out. Rise upward slightly
when turning left to the W and then sink slightly.
Turn the right palm out while sinking and
rerooting into the right leg.

IMAGES

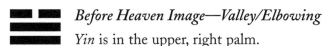 *Before Heaven Image—Valley/Elbowing*

Yin is in the upper, right palm.

Yang is in the left hip and left elbow.

Yang is in the left foot.

Elbowing occurs in the 1st movement. White Crane (an Elbowing technique) occurs in the 2nd movement.

Complementary Image—Mountain/Shouldering

It is from the Mountain that Wind flows down and gathers into the Valley. White Crane (Elbowing) must retain the intent of Pulling but rely on Shouldering. If no opportunity arises for Elbowing or Pulling, Shouldering is then the natural response and can be initiated in the 1st movement.

Eight Gates Image—Heaven/Warding-Off

The best stimulus for applying White Crane is when the opponent uses Warding-Off. Wind and Heaven rely on the support of Valley and Mountain. Heaven sustains the Mountain, and Wind seeks the Valley. When Elbowing and Shouldering fail, Pulling or Warding-Off can be used. Pulling aids Elbowing, and Warding-Off aids Shouldering. The Wind in the Valley moves up the Mountain and into Heaven.

After Heaven Image—Wind/Pulling

Wind moves through and is attracted by the Valley. Within White Crane there is Pulling, and it can be initiated in the transition from the 1st to the 2nd movement.

PHILOSOPHY

I Ching

When the wise man discovers what is correct, he will follow it. When he discovers errors, he corrects them.

Tao Te Ching

In seeking to expand, you must first contract. In seeking to be strong, you must first be weak. In wanting to receive, you must first give. This is called the profound wisdom of living.

T'ai Chi Ch'uan Classics

In practicing Sensing Hands, you must use the techniques of Adhering, Sticking, Joining, and Following with no letting go and with no resistance. If the opponent expands, you must contract; if he becomes forceful, you must weaken. When he attempts to take, you must give.

Brush Knee and Twist Step

Lou Hsi Yao Pu

After Heaven Image of **Sun**—*Wind (Pulling)*

TENTH POSTURE

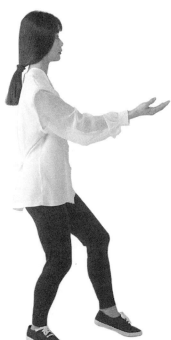

1st Movement

West—*Inhale*

Sink

Seated Tiger, Right

L Hand, *Lao Yin*—R Hand, *T'ai Yang*

Inhale as you sink your body slightly while bringing your right hand down, palm up, directly out from the midchest region.

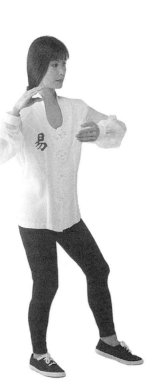

2nd Movement

Northwest—*Exhale*

Gazing-Right—Rise, Turn, Sink

Seated Tiger, Right

L Hand, *Chung Yin*—R Hand, *Shao Yang*

Exhale as you turn your body to the right, to the NW corner, while bringing your right hand across and turning it over (palm down) so that it is positioned level and out from the right ear. Simultaneously, the left hand and arm are brought upward and across to the right and end in a bow shape in front of the chest with the palm facing the body.

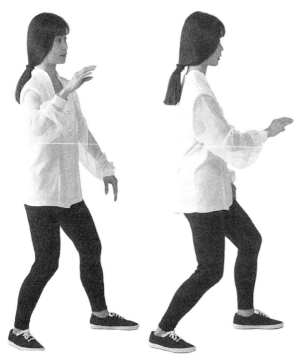

3rd Movement

West—*Inhale*

Advancing—Sink, Step, Shift

Looking-Left—Rise, Turn, Sink

Bow and Arrow, Left

L Hand, *Lao Yin*—R Hand, *T'ai Yin*

Inhale as you sink and step over and out (heel first) to the front with the left foot, keeping the waist and body to the NW. Simultaneously lower the left hand as if to brush it past the left knee while stepping. Next, put your left foot flat and shift your weight into the left leg. Then pick up your right toes and turn the waist and body left to face W, putting the right foot down pointing to the NW corner. While turning, lower the right hand so that it sits in front of the body, solar plexus level, with palm down and fingers pointing straight ahead.

4th Movement

West—*Exhale*

Advancing—Rise

Fixed-Rooting—Sink

Bow and Arrow, Left

L Hand, *Lao Yin*—R Hand, *Shao Yang*

Exhale as you rise off your rear leg (keeping both feet flat on the ground) while bringing the right arm slightly upward and out, with the palm facing out. The left hand is brought to the left side, palm facing back. Last, sink the entire body downward so that approximately 70 percent of the weight is in the forward (left) leg and 30 percent in the rear leg.

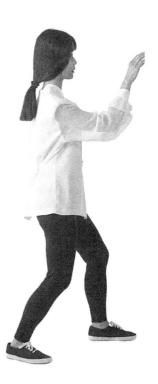

IMAGES

Before Heaven Image—Wind/Pulling

Yang is in the forward, right palm.

Yang is in the lower, left palm and right hip.

Yin is in the right foot.

Brush Knee (a Pulling technique) occurs in the transitions of the 2nd and 3rd movements. The Pulling takes place with the left hand.

Complementary Image—Thunder/Splitting

Wind is created by the movements within Earth. Thunder comes about from Winds meeting. Brush Knee (Pulling) must retain the intent of Rolling-Back but rely on Splitting. If no opportunity arises for Pulling or Rolling-Back, Splitting is then the natural response and can be initiated in the 1st and 3rd movement.

Eight Gates Image—Mountain/Shouldering

The best stimulus for applying Brush Knee is when the opponent uses Shouldering. Earth and Mountain rely on the support of Wind and Thunder. Thunder sustains the Mountain, and Wind seeks the Earth. When Brush Knee and Rolling-Back fail, Splitting or Shouldering can be used. Pulling aids Splitting, and Rolling-Back aids Shouldering.

After Heaven Image—Earth/Rolling-Back

Wind needs the resistance of the Earth in order to maintain its flow and movement. Within Brush Knee there is Rolling-Back, and it can be initiated in the transition from the 2nd to the 3rd movement.

PHILOSOPHY

I Ching

Returning is successful. Advancing and returning without any harm. Going to and fro is the Way.

Tao Te Ching

Tao is an endless circle, forever in a condition of return.

T'ai Chi Ch'uan Classics

When attacking above, you must not forget below. When striking to the left, you must pay attention to the right. When advancing, consider retreating. This is called T'ai Chi.

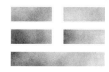

Playing the Lute

Shou Hui P'i Pa

After Heaven Image of **Chen**—*Thunder (Splitting)*

ELEVENTH POSTURE

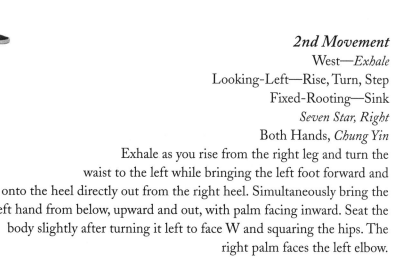

1st Movement
Northwest—*Inhale*
Advancing—Sink, Step
Gazing-Right—Shift, Turn, Sink
Immortal, Right
L Hand, *Lao Yin*—R Hand, *Chung Yin*
Inhale as you sink your weight entirely into the left leg, then step
straight forward with the right foot so that it is in line with the left
foot and the toes are pointed between the NW and N directions.
Simultaneously bring the right hand and arm down to the level of the
chest. Then immediately shift the weight to the right leg. Turn
the body slightly to the right and the right palm so that it
faces inward.

2nd Movement
West—*Exhale*
Looking-Left—Rise, Turn, Step
Fixed-Rooting—Sink
Seven Star, Right
Both Hands, *Chung Yin*
Exhale as you rise from the right leg and turn the
waist to the left while bringing the left foot forward and
onto the heel directly out from the right heel. Simultaneously bring the
left hand from below, upward and out, with palm facing inward. Seat the
body slightly after turning it left to face W and squaring the hips. The
right palm faces the left elbow.

IMAGES

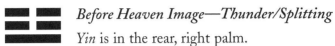

Before Heaven Image—Thunder/Splitting

Yin is in the rear, right palm.

Yin is in the front hip.

Yang is in the rear leg.

Playing the Guitar (Splitting) occurs in the 2nd movement.

Complementary Image—Wind/Pulling

Mountain stimulates the Wind, which creates the movements of Thunder. Playing the Guitar (Splitting) must retain the intent of Pulling but rely on Shouldering. If no opportunity arises for Splitting or Shouldering, Pulling is then the natural response and can be initiated in the 2nd movement.

Eight Gates Image—Earth/Rolling-Back

The best stimulus for applying Playing the Guitar is when the opponent uses Rolling-Back. Mountain and Earth rely on the support of Thunder and Wind. Thunder sustains the Mountain, and Wind seeks the Earth. When Playing the Guitar and Shouldering fail, Pulling or Rolling-Back can be used. Splitting aids Pulling, and Shouldering aids Rolling-Back.

After Heaven Image—Mountain/Shouldering

Mountains are created by Thunder. Within Playing the Guitar is Shouldering, and it can be initiated in the 1st movement.

PHILOSOPHY

I Ching

If there is nothing to advance toward, then withdrawing is good. If there is something to advance toward, then it should be done swiftly. Only the wise man can free himself from entanglements.

Tao Te Ching

The softest thing in the world can overcome the hardest. Such things seem to issue forth from nowhere.

T'ai Chi Ch'uan Classics

Entice him to Advance and Neutralize the incoming force until it is completely expended. Then use four ounces of energy to deflect the momentum of one thousand pounds.

Chop with Fist

P'ieh Ch'ui

After Heaven Image of K'an—*Water (Pressing)*

TWELFTH POSTURE

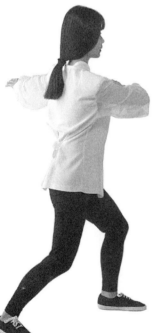

1st Movement
West—*Inhale*
Advancing—Sink, Step, Shift
Looking-Left—Turn, Sink
Immortal, Left
L Hand, *T'ai Yin*—R Hand, *T'ai Yin* (Fist)
Inhale as you sink the weight into the rear leg and step over and out with the left foot to be in an Immortal Stance (in which the left toes point NW), and then shift the weight into the left leg. Simultaneously bring both arms and hands, palm down, to midabdomen level with fingers pointing to the south. Then slightly turn left and form the right hand into a fist, palm down.

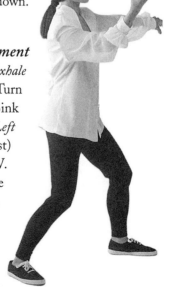

2nd Movement
Northwest—*Exhale*
Gazing-Right—Rise, Turn
Fixed-Rooting—Sink
Immortal, Left
L Hand, *T'ai Yin*—R Hand, *Shao Yin* (Fist)
Exhale as you begin turning your waist to the right to face NW. Simultaneously, with a slight forward motion of the right elbow, bring the right fist up and over to Chop.

IMAGES

 Before Heaven Images—Water/Pressing

Yin is in the right fist (Folding-Up).

Yang is in the left hip and the right elbow (Elbowing).

Yin is in the forward, left foot and the left palm (Pressing).

Chopping (a Pressing technique) occurs in the 2nd movement. Pressing occurs in the 1st movement.

Complementary Image—Fire/Pushing

Without Fire, Water cannot collect in the Valley. Chopping (Pressing) must retain the intent of Elbowing but rely on Pushing. If no opportunity arises for Chopping or Elbowing, Pushing is then the natural response and can be initiated at the end of the 1st movement.

Eight Gates Image—Thunder/Splitting

The best stimulus for applying Chopping is when the opponent uses Splitting. Valley and Thunder rely on the support of Water and Fire. Fire sustains Thunder, and Water seeks the Valley. When Chopping and Elbowing fail, Pushing or Splitting can be used. Pushing aids Splitting, and Pressing aids Elbowing.

After Heaven Images—Valley/Elbowing

Valleys provide Water with either the place to collect or flow through. Within Chopping there is Elbowing, and it can be initiated in the first part of the 2nd movement.

PHILOSOPHY

I Ching

In approaching others the wise man conceals his brightness, thus preserving his glory; not light, but shadows. First he may ascend to Heaven, then plunge to Earth.

Tao Te Ching

The Tao does not contend, but it forever wins. It receives responses without seeking them.

T'ai Chi Ch'uan Classics

The fundamental here is to forget the self and follow others. Most make the error of rejecting the near for what is distant.

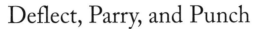

Deflect, Parry, and Punch

Pan Lan Ch'ui

After Heaven Image of Li—*Fire (Pushing)*

THIRTEENTH POSTURE

1st Movement

Southwest—*Inhale*

Looking-Left—Shift, Turn, Sink

Seven Star, Right

L Hand, *T'ai Yang*—R Hand, *T'ai Yin*

Inhale as you shift the weight into the rear leg, pick up the left-foot toes (keeping the heel on the floor), turn the body left to the SW corner, and then sink. Simultaneously bring the left arm and hand to be in front of the left hip with the palm facing upward; bring the right hand across to neck level with the palm facing down. The arms appear as if they are holding a ball.

2nd Movement

Southwest—*Exhale*

Advancing—Rise, Shift, Sink

Immortal, Left

L Hand, *T'ai Yang*—R Hand, *T'ai Yin*

Exhale as you place the left foot flat and shift the weight into the left leg, keeping the arms in the same position. The body still faces SW.

3rd Movement

West—*Inhale*

(Left Photo) Looking-Left—Sink, Turn

L Hand, *T'ai Yang*—R Hand, *T'ai Yin*

Twisting Dragon, Left

(Right Photo) Gazing-Right—Rise, Turn, Step, Sink

Seven Star, Left

L Hand, *Shao Yang*—R Hand, *Shao Yin* (Fist)

Inhale as you sink and turn your body toward the left (S). Then rise and begin turning back to the front (W) while stepping forward with the right foot onto the heel. Simultaneously bring the hands and arms around with this movement—with the right hand ending in a fist, palm up and parallel to the ground, and over the right toes. The left palm is placed out from the left ear, with palm facing out.

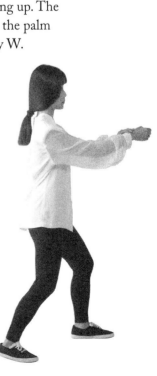

4th Movement

Northwest—*Exhale*

Gazing-Right—Shift, Turn, Sink

Twisting Dragon, Right

L Hand, *T'ai Yin*—R Hand, *Shao Yin* (Fist)

Exhale as you shift the weight to the right leg, turn the waist right to the NW, and sink the weight into the right leg. The left hand is lowered palm down until it's in line with and shoulders' width apart from the right forearm and hand.

5th Movement

West—*Inhale*

Advancing—Sink, Step, Shift

Looking-Left—Rise, Turn, Sink

Bow and Arrow, Left

L Hand, *Chung Yin*—R Hand, *Shao Yin* (Fist)

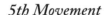

Inhale as you sink further into the right leg and step directly forward with the left foot. Then shift the weight into the left leg, pick up your right toes, and turn the waist left to the W, placing the toes down so that they point NW. Simultaneously draw the right fist back alongside the right hip, with the palm still facing up. The left hand moves out and across at chest level, with the palm facing inward and the fingertips pointing directly W.

6th Movement

West—*Exhale*

Advancing—Rise

Fixed-Rooting—Sink

Bow and Arrow, Left

L Hand, *Shao Yang*—R Hand, *Chung Yin* (Fist)

Exhale as you rise off your right leg (keeping the feet flat on the ground) and punch forward with the right hand. Simultaneously, as the punch is extending outward, bring the left arm inward and cup the left palm over the punching fist. As you conclude the punch, continue bringing the left arm inward until the fingertips rest on the right wrist. Sink the body slightly with 70 percent of the weight in the forward leg.

IMAGES

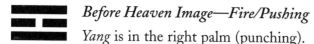 *Before Heaven Image—Fire/Pushing*

Yang is in the right palm (punching).

Yin is in the left hip and palm (parrying).

Yang is in the left foot (stepping in).

Deflect occurs in the 3rd movement. Parry occurs in the 4th and 5th movements. Punch occurs in the 6th movement. All three are Pushing techniques.

Complementary Image—Water/Pressing

Without Water all things dry and ignite (Thunder) into Fire. Parrying (Pushing) must retain the intent of Splitting, but rely on Pressing. If no opportunity arises for Parrying or Splitting, Pressing is then the natural response and can be initiated from the end of the 4th movement.

Eight Gates Image—Valley/Elbowing

The best stimulus for applying Parrying is when the opponent uses Elbowing (Chopping). Thunder and Valley rely on the support of Fire and Water. Thunder sustains Fire, and Valley attracts Water. When Parrying and Pressing fail, Splitting or Elbowing can be used. Splitting aids Pushing, and Elbowing aids Pressing.

After Heaven Image—Thunder/Splitting

Thunder creates Fire. Shaking brings about fires and earthquakes. Within Parrying there is Splitting, and it can be initiated in the 4th movement.

PHILOSOPHY

I Ching

The wise man's Mind-Intent for learning is limitless. He is boundless in both support and protection of others.

Tao Te Ching

In cultivating your mind, know how to delve into the abyss. In moving your body, know how to choose the right moment.

T'ai Chi Ch'uan Classics

The body turns and remains connected, moving neither too early or too late. Yield at the right moment.

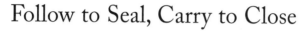

Follow to Seal, Carry to Close

*Ju Feng Shih Pi**

After Heaven Image of **Ch'ien**—*Heaven (Warding-Off)*

FOURTEENTH POSTURE

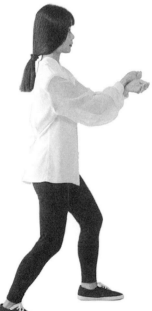

1st Movement
West—*Inhale*
Advancing—Rise, Sink
Bow and Arrow, Left
Both Hands, *T'ai Yang*
Inhale as you bring the body slightly upward. Simultaneously
lower the left hand and then slide it under the right wrist,
turning both palms to face upward as you do so. Slightly sink
the body as the palms are turning upward.

2nd Movement
West—*Exhale*
Withdrawing, Looking-Left—
Rise, Turn, Shift, Sink
Climbing a Mountain, Right
Both Hands, *T'ai Yin*
Exhale as you rise off the forward leg, make a slight turning
movement to the left while shifting back, and then sink
the weight into the right leg. Simultaneously turn both the right
and left palms down while drawing in the elbows toward the body,
keeping the forearms parallel to the floor.

---

*This posture is normally referred to as "Withdraw and Push" and in some cases "Apparent
Closure." These translations, however, are incorrect as they do not indicate the ideas of the intrinsic
energies of *Sealing* and *Closing*.

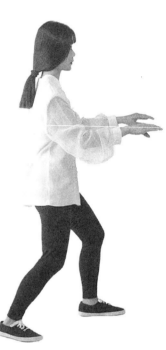

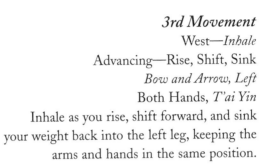

3rd Movement

West—*Inhale*

Advancing—Rise, Shift, Sink

Bow and Arrow, Left

Both Hands, *T'ai Yin*

Inhale as you rise, shift forward, and sink your weight back into the left leg, keeping the arms and hands in the same position.

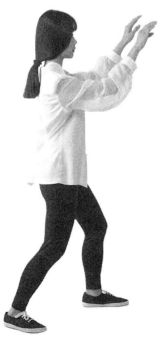

4th Movement

West—*Exhale*

Advancing—Rise

Fixed-Rooting—Sink

Bow and Arrow, Left

Both Hands, *Shao Yang*

Exhale as you rise off your rear leg (keeping the feet flat on the floor). Simultaneously bring the arms upward and out while slightly dropping the elbows so that the palms turn out. Last, sink the entire body downward so that approximately 70 percent of the weight is in the front leg and 30 percent in the rear leg.

IMAGES

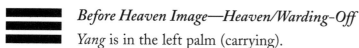 *Before Heaven Image—Heaven/Warding-Off*

Yang is in the left palm (carrying).
Yang is in the left hip and right arm (closing).
Yang is in left foot.

Follow to Seal occurs in the 1st and 2nd movements. Carry to Close occurs in the 3rd and 4th movements. This posture is sometimes referred to as Withdraw and Push, as that is what it appears to be. However, the characters for *Ju Feng Shih Pi* do not translate as Withdraw and Push, and this is actually a misleading interpretation considering that its true application incorporates Warding-Off energy.

Complementary Image—Earth/Rolling-Back

If there is no Fire (sun), the light of Heaven (sky) cannot sustain the Earth. Sealing and Closing (Warding-Off) must retain the intent of Pushing, but rely on Rolling-Back. If no opportunity arises for Sealing and Closing or Pushing, Rolling-Back is then the natural response and can be initiated from the end of the 1st and 2nd movements.

Eight Gates Image—Water/Pressing

The best stimulus for applying Sealing and Closing is when the opponent uses Pressing. Fire and Water rely on the support of Heaven and Water. Heaven sustains Earth, and Fire harmonizes Water. When Sealing and Closing and Rolling-Back fail, Pushing or Pressing can be used. Warding-Off aids Pushing, and Rolling-Back aids Pressing.

After Heaven Image—Fire/Pushing

Fire (brightness and light) are the qualities of Heaven. Within Sealing and Closing there is Pushing, and it can be initiated in the 2nd and 4th movements.

PHILOSOPHY

I Ching

The wise man restrains himself in order to avoid dangers. He seeks neither praise nor gain.

Tao Te Ching

It is because you do not contend that you will not be at fault.

T'ai Chi Ch'uan Classics

T'ai Chi is second to none because it does not contend.

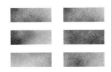

Crossing Hands

Shih Tsu Shou

After Heaven Image of K'un—Earth (Rolling-Back)

FIFTEENTH POSTURE

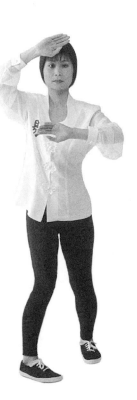

1st Movement
West—*Inhale*
Withdrawing—Rise, Shift, Sink
Climbing a Mountain, Right
Both Hands, *T'ai Yin*
Inhale as you rise, shift back, and sink your weight into the rear leg. Simultaneously lower both hands and arms to be in line with the shoulders.

2nd Movement
North—*Exhale*
Gazing-Right—Rise, Turn, Sink
Eight Shape, Right
Both Hands, *Chung Yang*
Exhale as you pick up the toes of your left foot, and pivot on the heel while turning your waist and body left toward the N. Put the left foot down so that the side of the foot is in line with the front (N) and sink the weight into the right leg. Simultaneously, bring the right palm to face outward at forehead level. The left hand moves so that the palm faces out at lower-neck level.

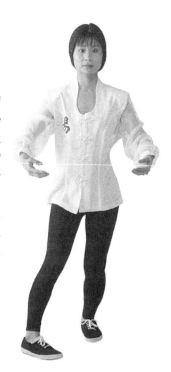

3rd Movement

North—*Inhale*

Withdrawing—Rise, Shift, Sink

Eight Shape, Left

Both Hands, *T'ai Yang*

Inhale as you shift and sink your weight back into the left foot. Simultaneously circle both hands outward and down, as if scooping something upward. Both hands end palm up at lower-abdomen level.

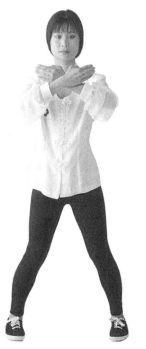

4th Movement

North—*Exhale*

Withdrawing—Rise, Step

Fixed-Rooting—Sink

Riding a Horse, Left

Both Hands, *Shao Yin*

Exhale as you raise the body upward, pick up the right heel, and draw the foot back to move the body into Riding a Horse Stance. Simultaneously, the hands move upward, crossing at the wrists, right hand on the outside, until the palms face the body at lower-neck level. Sink the body slightly at the end of this movement.

IMAGES

Before Heaven Image—Earth/Rolling-Back

Yin is in the right palm.

Yin is in the right hip.

Yin is in the right foot.

Rolling-Back occurs in the 2nd movement. Crossing Hands (a Rolling-Back technique) occurs in the 3rd and 4th movements.

Complementary Image—Heaven/Warding-Off

Heaven is but an archetype of Earth. Without Water on the Earth, Heaven would have nothing on which to reflect its likeness. Rolling-Back must retain the intent of Pressing but rely on Warding-Off. If no opportunity arises for Crossing Hands (Rolling-Back) or Pressing, Warding-Off is then the natural response and can be initiated from the 3rd and 4th movements.

Eight Gates Image—Fire/Pushing

The best stimulus for applying Crossing Hands is when the opponent uses Pushing. Water and Fire rely on the support of Earth and Heaven. Earth supports Water, and Heaven relies on Fire. When Crossing Hands and Warding-Off fail, Pressing or Pushing can be used. Rolling-Back aids Pressing, and Warding-Off aids Pushing.

After Heaven Image—Water/Pressing

Water sustains and collects on the Earth. Within Crossing Hands there is Pressing, and it can be initiated in the 3rd and 4th movements.

PHILOSOPHY

I Ching

The wise man is constantly reexamining himself, and so forever improves upon his own nature.

Tao Te Ching

Those who know others are wise. Those who know themselves are illumined. Those who master others have strength. Those who master themselves have power.

T'ai Chi Ch'uan Classics

Through self-mastery you will gradually apprehend interpreting and you will reach a state of spiritual illumination. The opponent does not know you, but you alone know him.

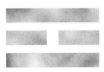

Conclusion of T'ai Chi

Ho T'ai Chi

After Heaven Image of Li—*Fire (Pushing)*

SIXTEENTH POSTURE

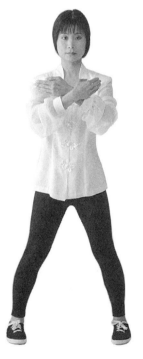

1st Movement
North—*Inhale*
Rise
Seated Horse
Both Hands, *Shao Yin*
Inhale as you raise the body upward and place equal weight on both legs.

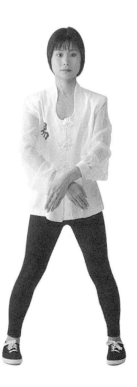

2nd Movement
North—*Exhale*
Sink
Seated Horse
Both Hands, *Lao Yin*
Exhale as you sink the body. Slightly lower the hands, with hands still crossed, down to lower-abdomen level. The palms still face the body.

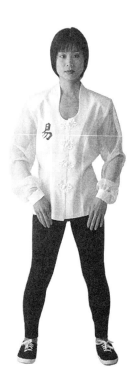

3rd Movement

North—*Inhale*
Rise
Seated Horse
Both Hands, *Lao Yin*
Inhale as you slightly raise the body and
separate the hands so that they rest on
the front of the thighs.

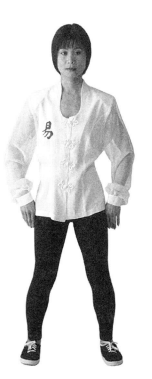

4th Movement

North—*Exhale*
Sink
Seated Horse
Both Hands, *Lao Yin*
Exhale as you seat the body. Bring the hands over
to the sides of each thigh, with thumbs lightly
touching the thighs, and slightly press
the elbows forward.

IMAGES

 Before Heaven Image—Fire/Pushing

Yang is in both palms.

Yin is in the abdomen.

Yang is in both feet.

Pushing here is symbolic of the breath and *ch'i* rising and circulating freely throughout the body.

Complementary Image—Water/Pressing

When Water is over Fire the vapors of *ch'i* begin to move, and the Elixir of Immortality is being formed within the body. This is like the heat within the Earth, warming all the fluids so they may move and nourish all things. Here the Fire is successfully pushing the *ch'i* throughout the body (through the bloodstream and *ch'i* meridians).

Eight Gates Image—Valley/Elbowing

The T'ai Chi Conclusion Posture is like a vibration (Thunder) striking in the Valley to move and stimulate the Fire and Water into their correct positions. Fire is now below Water. Fire is being pushed up from the Valley by Thunder (the movements). The best stimulus for Fire is to contain it in the Valley to build it.

After Heaven Image—Thunder/Splitting

Heaven is revealed by light (Fire). When the *ch'i* is moved (Thunder) in the body, light is produced in the head (Heaven).

PHILOSOPHY

I Ching

The wise man stands firm, without ever having to change direction.

Tao Te Ching

Returning is the movement of Tao. Receptivity is the way in which the Tao is used.

T'ai Chi Ch'uan Classics

To adhere is to receive; to receive is to adhere. *Yin* is not separate from *yang; yang* is not separate from *yin.*

Wu Chi Position

Wu Chi Shih

Stand erect, with feet held at shoulders' width distance apart and hands held in *Lao Yin* position. Suspend the head, gaze levelly, place the tongue against the palate, and focus the attention into the *tan-t'ien*. Perform three or more complete breaths before ending.

Note: When you become proficient in performing these sixteen postures you should further develop your practice by teaching yourself how to practice the form to the opposite, or left, side. This will then strengthen and bring about complete harmony within the body and mind.

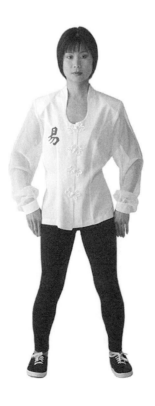

BEFORE HEAVEN FORM POSTURE
MOVEMENTS SUMMARY

Wu Chi *Position*

N

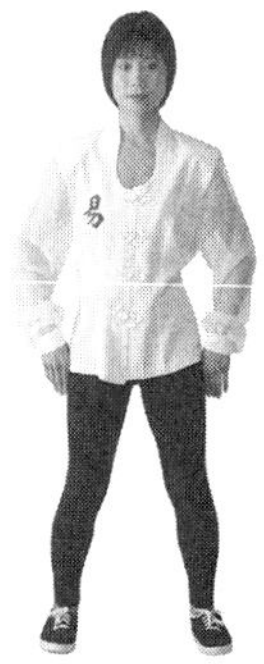

Beginning T'ai Chi
1st Movement
N

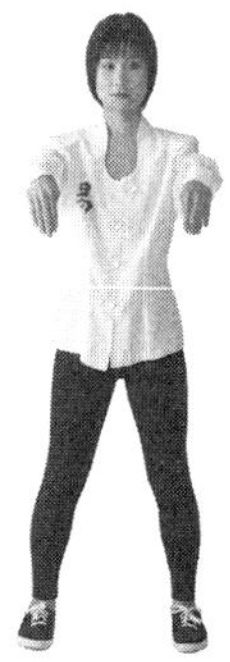

2nd Movement
N

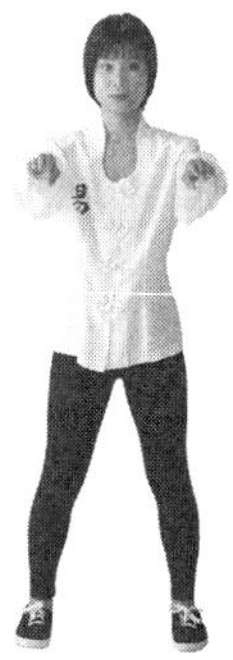

3rd Movement
N

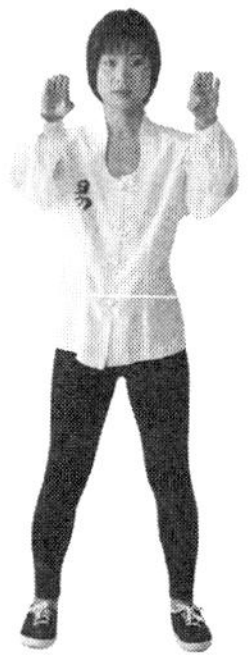

4th Movement
N

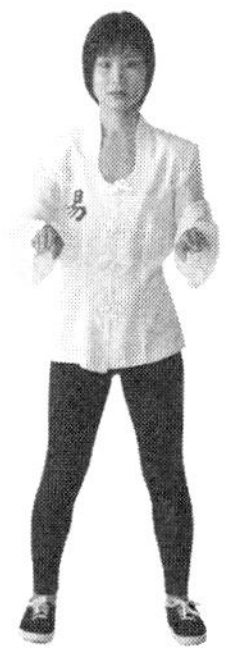

5th Movement
N

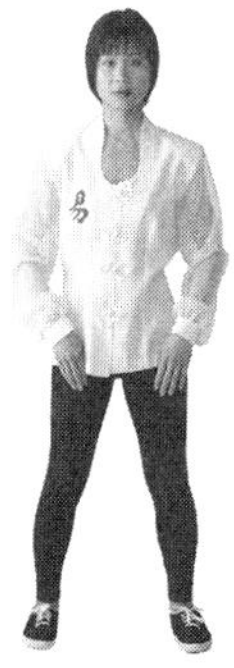

6th Movement
N

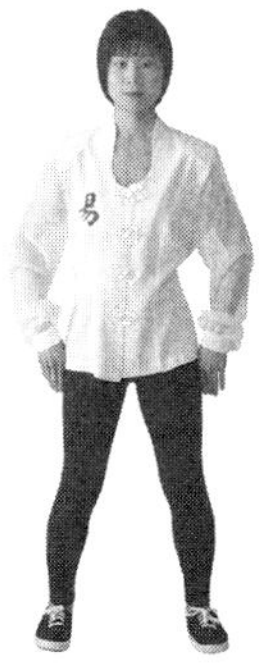

Warding-Off, Left
1st Movement
NE

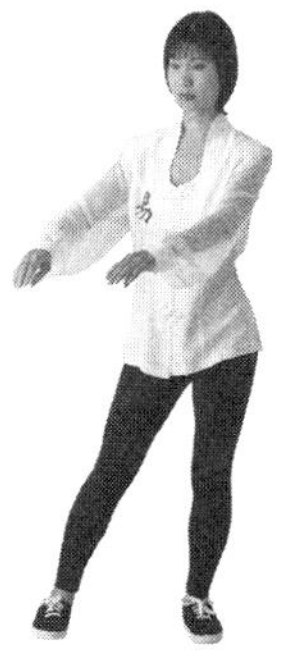

2nd Movement
E

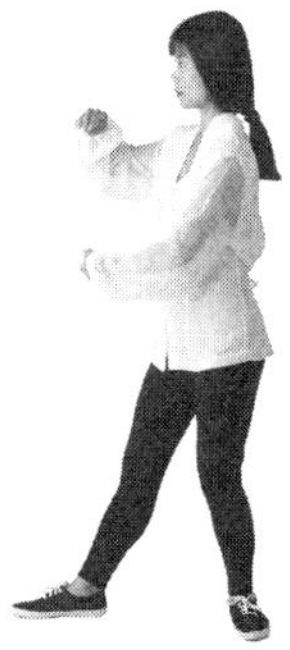

3rd Movement
E

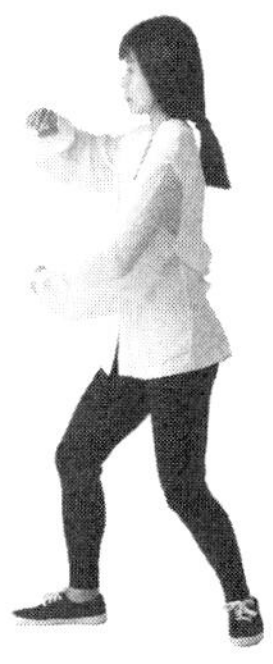

4th Movement
NE

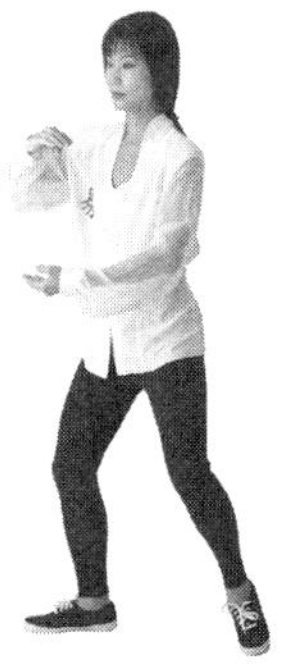

5th Movement
N

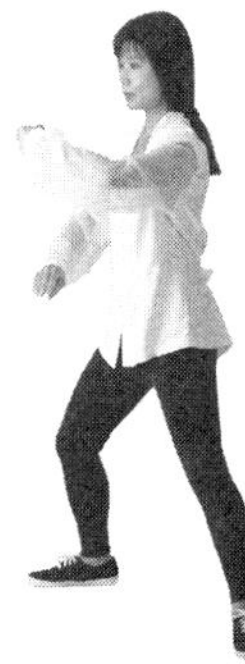

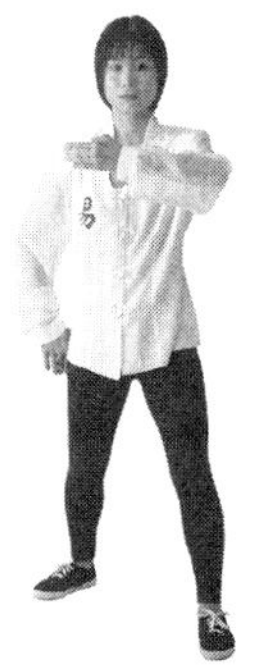

6th Movement
N

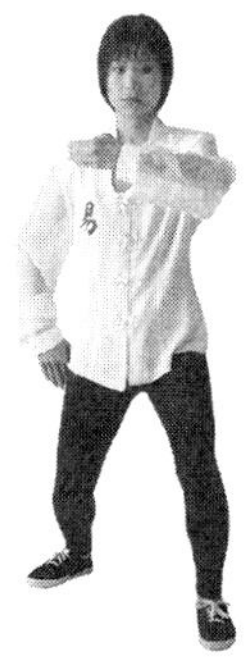

Warding-Off, Right

1st Movement	2nd Movement	3rd Movement	4th Movement
N	NE	E	E

Rolling-Back

1st Movement	2nd Movement	3rd Movement	4th Movement
SE	E	E	NE

Pressing

1st Movement	2nd Movement	3rd Movement	4th Movement
N	E	E	E

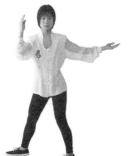
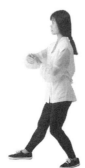
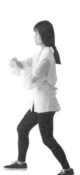
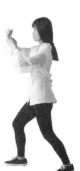

Pushing

1st Movement E	2nd Movement E	3rd Movement E	4th Movement E

Single Whip

1st Movement E	2nd Movement N	3rd Movement NE	4th Movement NW

5th Movement W	6th Movement W	*Lifting Hands* 1st Movement NW	2nd Movement N

Shouldering

1st Movement	2nd Movement
N	N

White Crane Spreads Wings

1st Movement	2nd Movement
NW	W

Brush Knee and Twist Step

1st Movement	2nd Movement	3rd Movement	4th Movement
W	NW	W	W

Playing the Guitar

1st Movement	2nd Movement
W	W

Chop with Fist

1st Movement	2nd Movement
W	NW

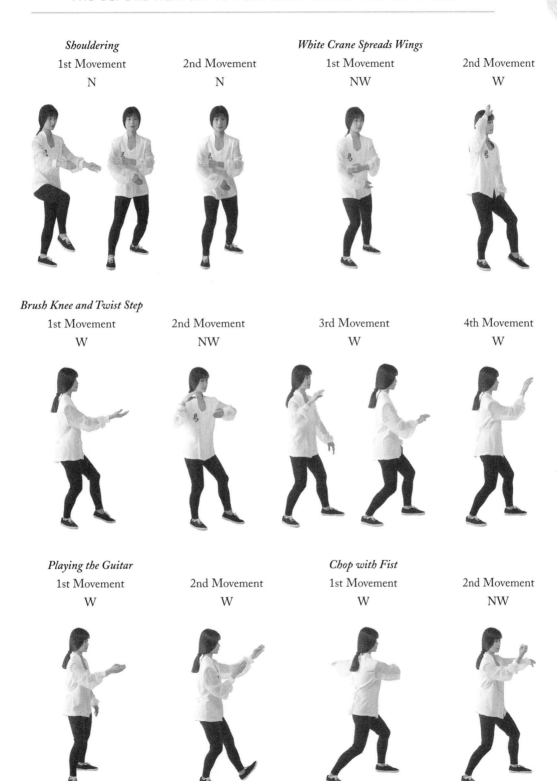

Deflect, Parry, and Punch

1st Movement	2nd Movement	3rd Movement
SW	SW	W

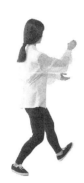
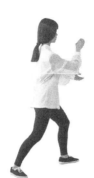
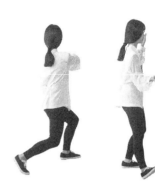

4th Movement	5th Movement	6th Movement
NW	W	W

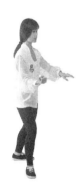
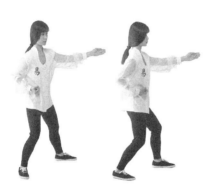
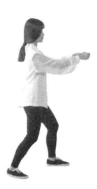

Follow to Seal, Carry to Close

1st Movement	2nd Movement	3rd Movement	4th Movement
W	W	W	W

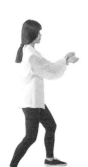
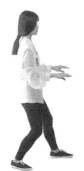
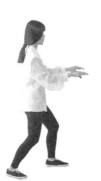
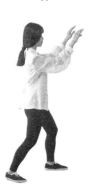

Crossing Hands

1st Movement	2nd Movement	3rd Movement	4th Movement
W	N	N	N

Conclusion of T'ai Chi

1st Movement	2nd Movement	3rd Movement	4th Movement
N	N	N	N

Wu Chi *Position*

N

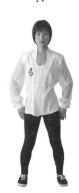

PART IV

The After Heaven Form

Although the form instructions and detailed explanations of the construction of the After Heaven 64-Posture I Ching T'ai Chi Form will appear in a future publication, I present the charts following to demonstrate the basis for constructing the 64-Posture Form according to the I Ching hexagrams (six-lined images).

16 Arranging the Images of the Sixty-Four Postures

The 64-Posture I Ching T'ai Chi Form is comprised of eight sections with eight postures in each section. The sections follow the natural sequence of the Before Heaven arrangement, determined by the lower three-lined image. The form moves in a sequence of eight postures of which Heaven is the lower image, to eight postures of which Valley is the lower image, to eight postures of which Fire is the lower image, and so on. The upper three-lined images are arranged in a similar fashion to the Before Heaven 16-Posture Form, wherein the 16th Posture image is the Complement of the 1st Posture image, and the 15th image is the Complement of the 2nd image, the 14th to the 3rd, the 13th to the 4th, and so forth.

Each sequence of eight images in the 64-Posture Form likewise follows a similar pattern of working in on itself through its complementary images. The arrangement of each sequence of the upper images is described below and can be seen in the charts and form arrangements in this section of the book.

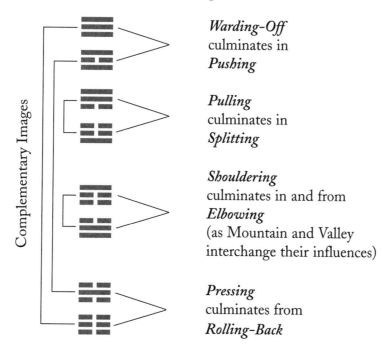

Warding-Off
culminates in
Pushing

Pulling
culminates in
Splitting

Shouldering
culminates in and from
Elbowing
(as Mountain and Valley
interchange their influences)

Pressing
culminates from
Rolling-Back

203

CIRCULAR CHART OF THE 64 POSTURES
(Heaven)

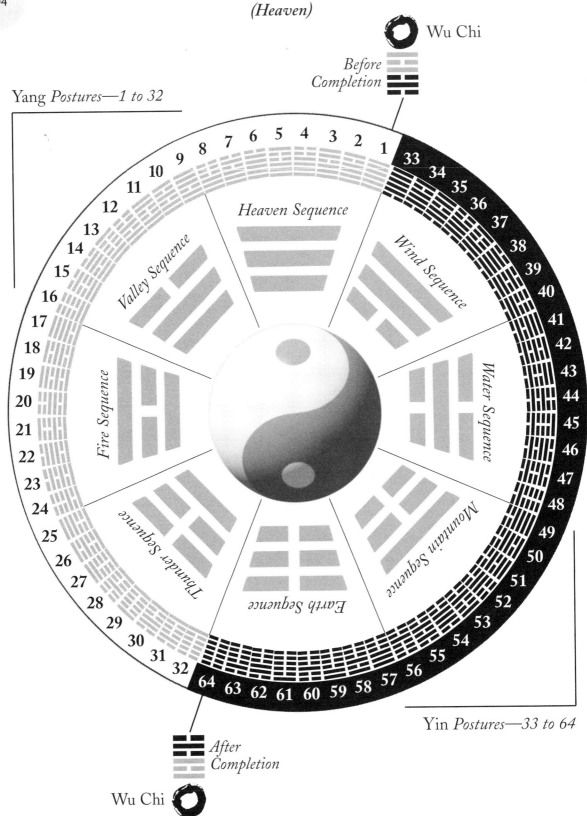

Wu Chi

Before Completion

Yang *Postures—1 to 32*

Heaven Sequence

Valley Sequence

Wind Sequence

Water Sequence

Fire Sequence

Mountain Sequence

Thunder Sequence

Earth Sequence

Yin *Postures—33 to 64*

After Completion

Wu Chi

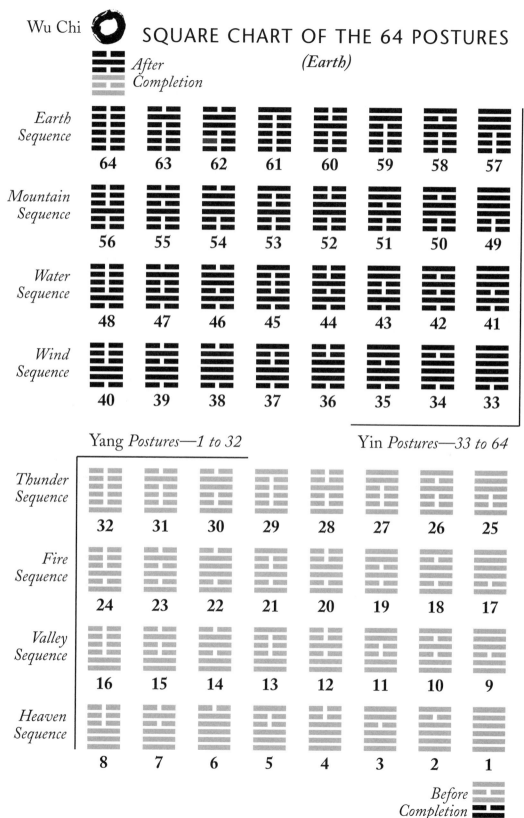

Wu Chi

SQUARE CHART OF THE 64 POSTURES
(Earth)

After Completion

Earth Sequence
64 63 62 61 60 59 58 57

Mountain Sequence
56 55 54 53 52 51 50 49

Water Sequence
48 47 46 45 44 43 42 41

Wind Sequence
40 39 38 37 36 35 34 33

Yang *Postures—1 to 32*   Yin *Postures—33 to 64*

Thunder Sequence
32 31 30 29 28 27 26 25

Fire Sequence
24 23 22 21 20 19 18 17

Valley Sequence
16 15 14 13 12 11 10 9

Heaven Sequence
8 7 6 5 4 3 2 1

Before Completion

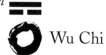 Wu Chi

LINEAR CHART OF THE 64 POSTURES
(Man)

Wu Chi ⭕ Yang *Postures—1 to 32*

Before Completion

Heaven Sequence

Fire Sequence

Wind Sequence

Mountain Sequence

1　17　33　49

2　18　34　50

3　19　35　51

4　20　36　52

5　21　37　53

6　22　38　54

7　23　39　55

8　24　40　56

9　25　41　57

10　26　42　58

11　27　43　59

12　28　44　60

13　29　45　61

14　30　46　62

15　31　47　63

16　32　48　64

Valley Sequence

Thunder Sequence

Water Sequence

Earth Sequence

After Completion

Yin *Postures—33 to 64*　Wu Chi

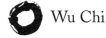

THE AFTER HEAVEN
64-POSTURE
I CHING T'AI CHI FORM

(Hou T'ien T'ai Chi)

*64-Posture T'ai Chi According to the Interaction
of the Sixty-Four Images*

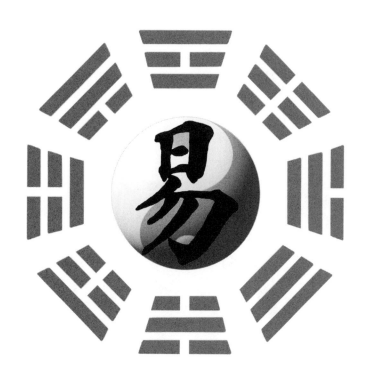

YANG POSTURES 1–8,
T'AI YANG (HEAVEN) SEQUENCE

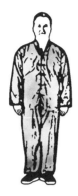

Wu Chi
North

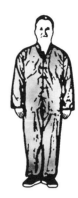

Preparation
Fire over Water
North
2 Counts

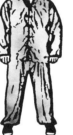
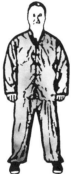

Posture 1

Beginning T'ai Chi
Heaven Style
North
6 Counts

Posture 2

Grasp the Bird's Tail, #1
Fire Style
East
22 Counts

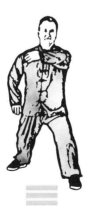

Warding-Off, Left

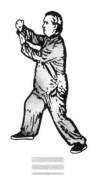

Warding-Off, Right

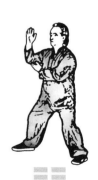

Rolling-Back

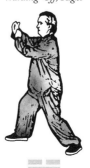

Pressing

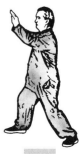

Pushing

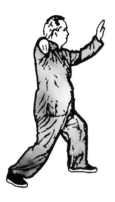

Posture 3

Single Whip, #1
Wind Style
West
6 Counts

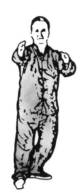

Posture 4

Lifting Hands, #1
Thunder Style
North
2 Counts

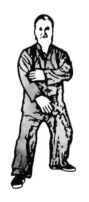

Posture 5

Shouldering, #1
Mountain Style
North
2 Counts

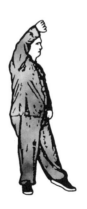

Posture 6

White Crane
Spreads Wings, #1
Valley Style
West, 2 Counts

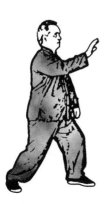

Posture 7

Brush Left Knee
and Twist Step, #1
Water Style
West, 4 Counts

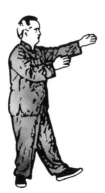

Posture 8

Playing the Guitar
Earth Style
West
2 Counts

YANG POSTURES 9–16,
SHAO YANG (VALLEY) SEQUENCE

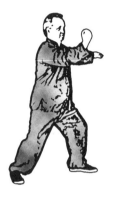

Posture 9

Chop with Fist
Heaven Style
Northwest
2 Counts

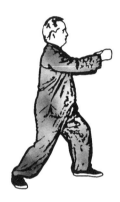

Posture 10

Deflect, Parry,
and Punch, #1
Fire Style
West, 6 Counts

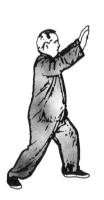

Posture 11

Follow to Seal,
Carry to Close, #1
Wind Style
West, 4 Counts

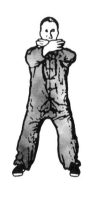

Posture 12

Crossing Hands, #1
Thunder Style
North
4 Counts

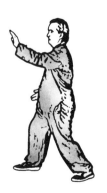

Posture 13

Embrace Tiger,
Return to Mountain
Mountain Style
Southeast, 4 Counts

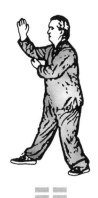

Posture 14

**Grasp the
Bird's Tail, #2**
*Valley Style
Northeast, 12 Counts*

Rolling-Back

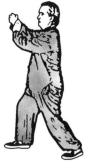

Pressing

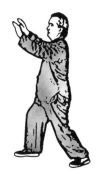

Pushing

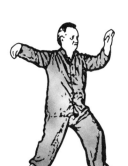

Posture 15

**Slanting
Single Whip**
*Water Style
Northwest, 6 Counts*

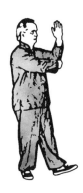

Posture 16

**Punch Under
the Elbow**
*Earth Style
West, 6 Counts*

YANG POSTURES 17–24,
CHUNG YANG (FIRE) SEQUENCE

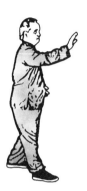

Posture 17

**Retreat to Chase
the Monkey Away**
*Heaven Style
West, 12 Counts*

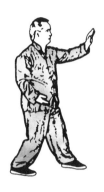

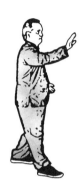

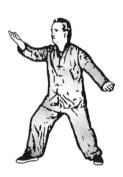

Posture 18

Flying Aslant
*Fire Style
Northeast
4 Counts*

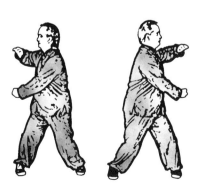

Posture 19

**Hands Waving
in Clouds, #1**
*Wind Style
Northwest, 4 Counts*

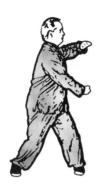

Posture 20

Hands Waving in Clouds, #2
Thunder Style
Northwest, 8 Counts

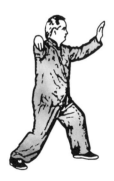

Posture 21

Single Whip, #2
Mountain Style
West
4 Counts

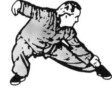

Posture 22

Glide Down Like Snake, #1
Valley Style
West, 4 Counts

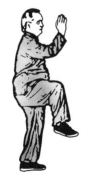

Posture 23

Golden Rooster Stands on Left Leg
Water Style
West, 2 Counts

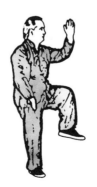

Posture 24

Golden Rooster Stands on Right Leg
Earth Style
West, 2 Counts

YANG POSTURES 25–32,
LAO YANG (THUNDER) SEQUENCE

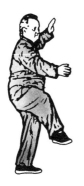

Posture 25

**Separate Hands,
Kicking with
Right Foot**
*Heaven Style
Northwest, 6 Counts*

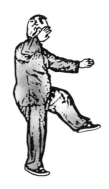

Posture 26

**Separate Hands,
Kicking with
Left Foot**
*Fire Style
Southwest, 6 Counts*

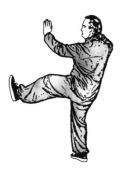

Posture 27

**Turn and Strike
with Heel**
*Wind Style
East, 4 Counts*

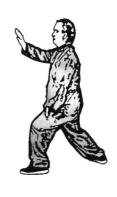

Posture 28

**Brush Left Knee
and Twist Step, #2**
*Thunder Style
East, 4 Counts*

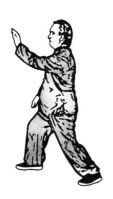

Posture 29

**Brush Right Knee
and Twist Step**
*Mountain Style
East, 4 Counts*

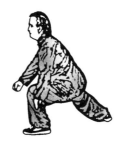

Posture 30

Punch Downward
*Valley Style
East
4 Counts*

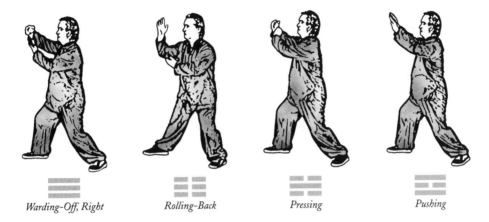

Warding-Off, Right   *Rolling-Back*   *Pressing*   *Pushing*

Posture 31

Grasp the Bird's Tail, #3
Water Style
East
16 Counts

Posture 32

Single Whip, #3
Earth Style
West
6 Counts

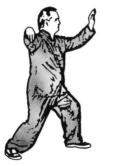

YIN POSTURES 33–40,
LAO YIN (WIND) SEQUENCE

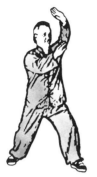

Posture 33

**Jade Maiden Weaves
at Shuttles, #1**
Heaven Style
Northeast, 6 Counts

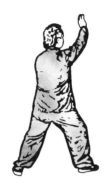

Posture 34

**Jade Maiden Weaves
at Shuttles, #2**
Fire Style
Northwest, 6 Counts

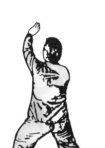

Posture 35

**Jade Maiden Weaves
at Shuttles, #3**
Wind Style
Southwest, 6 Counts

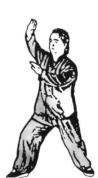

Posture 36

**Jade Maiden Weaves
at Shuttles, #4**
Thunder Style
Southeast, 6 Counts

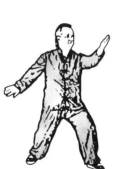
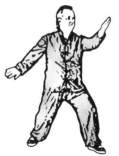

Posture 37

**Parting Wild
Horse's Mane, Left**
Mountain Style
Northwest, 4 Counts

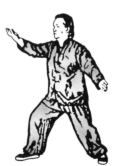

Posture 38

**Parting Wild
Horse's Main, Right**
Valley Style
Northeast, 4 Counts

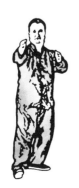

Posture 39

Lifting Hands, #2
Water Style
North
2 Counts

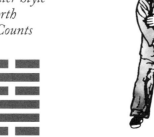

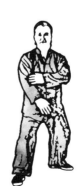
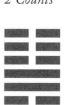

Posture 40

Shouldering, #2
Earth Style
North
2 Counts

YANG POSTURES 41–48, CHUNG YIN (WATER) SEQUENCE

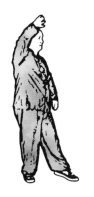

Posture 41
White Crane Spreads Wings, #2
Heaven Style
West, 2 Counts

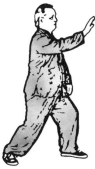

Posture 42
Brush Left Knee and Twist Step, #3
Fire Style
West, 4 Counts

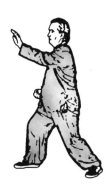

Posture 43
Get Needle off Sea Bottom
Wind Style
West, 4 Counts

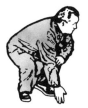

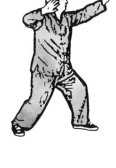

Posture 44
Penetrate Like Fan to the Back
Thunder Style
West, 4 Counts

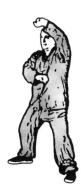

Posture 45
Turn and Chop with Fist
Mountain Style
East, 4 Counts

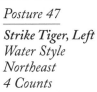

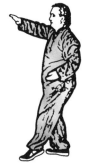

Posture 46
High Pat on Horse
Valley Style
East
4 Counts

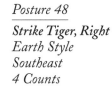

Posture 47
Strike Tiger, Left
Water Style
Northeast
4 Counts

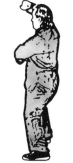

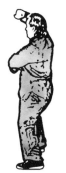

Posture 48
Strike Tiger, Right
Earth Style
Southeast
4 Counts

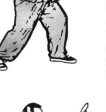

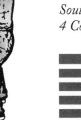

YIN POSTURES 49–56,
SHAO YIN (MOUNTAIN) SEQUENCE

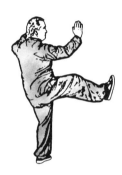

Posture 49

**Turn to Push
and Kick
with Heel**
*Heaven Style
West, 4 Counts*

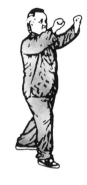

Posture 50

**Double Winds
Strike the Ears**
*Fire Style
Northwest, 4 Counts*

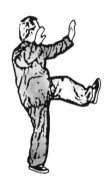

Posture 51

**Raise the Body
and Kick**
*Wind Style
Southwest, 4 Counts*

Posture 52

Thrusting Hand
*Thunder Style
West
4 Counts*

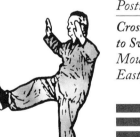

Posture 53

**Crossing Hands
to Sweep Lotuses**
*Mountain Style
East, 4 Counts*

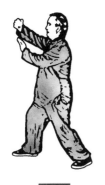

Warding-Off, Right

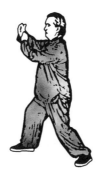

Rolling-Back

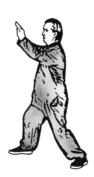

Pressing

Pushing

Posture 54

Grasp the Bird's Tail, #4
Valley Style
East
16 Counts

Posture 55

Single Whip, #4
Water Style
West
6 Counts

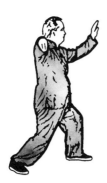

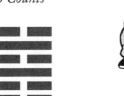

Posture 56

**Glide Down Like
Snake, #2**
Earth Style
West, 4 Counts

YIN POSTURES 57—64,
T'AI YIN (EARTH) SEQUENCE

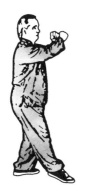

Posture 57

**Step Forward
to Seven Star**
Heaven Style
West, 2 Counts

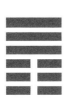

Posture 58

**Retreat to Ride
the Tiger**
Fire Style
West, 2 Counts

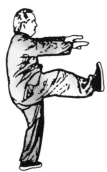

Posture 59

**Turn Body to
Sweep Lotuses**
Wind Style
West, 6 Counts

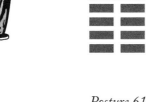

Posture 60

**Bend Bow to
Shoot the Tiger**
Thunder Style
Southwest, 4 Counts

Posture 61

**Deflect, Parry,
and Punch, #2**
Mountain Style
West, 6 Counts

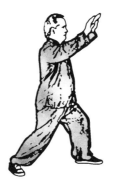

Posture 62

**Follow to Seal,
Carry to Close, #2**
Valley Style
West, 4 Counts

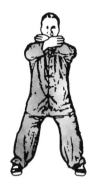

Posture 63

Crossing Hands, #2
Water Style
North
4 Counts

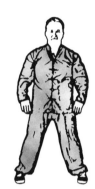

Posture 64

Conclusion
of T'ai Chi
Earth Style
North, 4 Counts

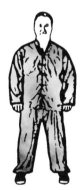

Completion
Water over Fire
North

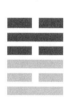

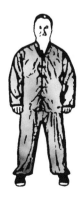

Wu Chi
North

After Heaven Sequence
64-POSTURE I CHING T'AI CHI FORM

Wu Chi Position

Preparation

Fire over
Water

Yang *Postures—1 to 32*

	Heaven		Fire
1. Beginning T'ai Chi		17. Retreat to Chase the Monkey Away	
2. Grasp the Bird's Tail, #1		18. Flying Aslant	
3. Single Whip, #1		19. Hands Waving in Clouds, #1	
4. Lifting Hands, #1		20. Hands Waving in Clouds, #2	
5. Shouldering, #1		21. Single Whip, #2	
6. White Crane Spreads Wings, #1		22. Glide Down Like Snake, #1	
7. Brush Left Knee and Twist Step, #1		23. Golden Rooster Stands on Left Leg	
8. Playing the Guitar		24. Golden Rooster Stands on Right Leg	

	Valley		Thunder
9. Chop with Fist		25. Separate Hands, kicking with Right Foot	
10. Deflect, Parry, and Punch, #1		26. Separate Hands, kicking with Left Foot	
11. Follow to Seal, Carry to Close, #1		27. Turn and Strike with Heel	
12. Crossing Hands, #1		28. Brush Left Knee and Twist Step, #2	
13. Embrace Tiger, Return to Mountain		29. Brush Right Knee and Twist Step	
14. Grasp the Bird's Tail, #2		30. Punch Downward	
15. Slanting Single Whip		31. Grasp the Bird's Tail, #3	
16. Punch Under the Elbow		32. Single Whip, #3	

	Wind		Mountain
33. Jade Maiden Weaves at Shuttles, #1		49. Turn to Push and Kick with Heel	
34. Jade Maiden, #2		50. Double Winds Strike the Ears	
35. Jade Maiden, #3		51. Raise the Body and Kick	
36. Jade Maiden, #4		52. Thrusting Hand	
37. Parting Wild Horse's Mane, Left		53. Crossing Hands to Sweep Lotuses	
38. Parting Wild Horse's Mane, Right		54. Grasp the Bird's Tail, #4	
39. Lifting Hands, #2		55. Single Whip, #4	
40. Shouldering, #2		56. Glide Down Like Snake, #2	

	Water		Earth
41. White Crane Spreads Wings, #2		57. Step Forward to Seven Star	
42. Brush Left Knee and Twist Step, #3		58. Retreat to Ride the Tiger	
43. Get Needle off Sea Bottom		59. Turn Body to Sweep Lotuses	
44. Penetrate Like Fan to the Back		60. Bend Bow to Shoot the Tiger	
45. Turn and Chop with Fist		61. Deflect, Parry, and Punch, #2	
46. High Pat on Horse		62. Follow to Seal, Carry to Close, #2	
47. Strike Tiger, Left		63. Crossing Hands, #2	
48. Strike Tiger, Right		64. Conclusion of T'ai Chi	

Completion   *Water* over *Fire*

Wu Ch

About the Author

n 1979, as a resident of Ju Lai Ssu monastery at the City of Ten-Thousand Buddhas in Talmage, California, Stuart began learning the Chinese language and studying Buddhist philosophy, taking formal refuge in Buddhism from Ch'an Master Hsuan Hua.

In 1982 the famous T'ai Chi Ch'uan master Tung-tsai Liang (presently 100 years old) invited Stuart to live and study with him at his home in St. Cloud, Minnesota. Stuart was the only student ever granted this honor. While staying in Master Liang's home for over six years, Stuart studied both T'ai Chi Ch'uan and the Chinese language under Master Liang's tutelage. Since then Stuart has traveled extensively throughout the United States with Master Liang, assisting him in teaching. Stuart has also taught in Canada, Hong Kong, and Indonesia, and has traveled throughout Asia. He has also studied massage in both Taiwan and Indonesia.

Stuart presently lives in northern California, where he writes about Asia-related subjects and teaches.

If you wish to contact him you may do so by forwarding mail to the publisher or e-mailing him at yitaichi@mediaone.net.

Books of Related Interest

THE COMPLETE I CHING
The Definitive Translation by the Taoist Master Alfred Huang

THE NUMEROLOGY OF THE I CHING
A Sourcebook of Symbols, Structures, and Traditional Wisdom
by Master Alfred Huang

MARTIAL ARTS TEACHING TALES OF POWER AND PARADOX
Freeing the Mind, Focusing Chi, and Mastering the Self
by Pascal Fauliot

THE PEACEFUL WAY
A Children's Guide to the Traditions of the Martial Arts
by Claudio Iedwab and Roxanne Standefer

THE SPIRITUAL FOUNDATIONS OF AIKIDO
by William Gleason

SHARP SPEAR, CRYSTAL MIRROR
Martial Arts in Women's Lives
by Stephanie T. Hoppe

I CHING FOR TEENS
Take Charge of Your Destiny with the Ancient Chinese Oracle
by Julie Tallard Johnson

TAO AND T'AI CHI KUNG
by Robert C. Sohn

Inner Traditions • Bear & Company
P.O. Box 388
Rochester, VT 05767
1-800-246-8648
www.InnerTraditions.com
Or contact your local bookseller